Delivering

DOCTOR MOTHER ADVOCATE

Kellie Lease Stecher, MD

Fisher King Publishing

Fisher King Publishing
The Old Barn
York Road
Thirsk
YO7 3AD
England

fisherkingpublishing.co.uk

Cover photograph by Dahli Durley

For Joseph and Addison, my children,
whom I love with my whole heart.
I work on these social justice and
healthcare issues so that they can work
and live in a healthier culture.

Dedication

This book is dedicated to those who love with their entire hearts. It is dedicated to the women in the world who have non-disclosure agreements and non-disparagement agreements. I realize it is an eviscerating pain to not be able to control your own life story. It is important for me to say to you all; I see you, I hear you, I walk with you, and I will fight for you and improved culture in whatever field you are in and however you choose to live your life. Many women feel pressured into signing the contracts because they fear the other person.

To my haters who might listen; without you I would never have found my strength and passions in life. To the people who hated my honesty, authenticity and the fact that I told my story without fear. Every stumble made me more motivated and resolved to make changes in this world.

To my patients and the community in which I reside. We are Minnesota strong. Every day you inspire me to do my job and look forward to helping you. It is my honor to be able to take care of you and your families.

To the amazing, strong, and fierce women who have paved the way for all of us; Supreme Court Justice Ruth Bader Ginsberg and Elizabeth Blackwell, the first female physician to receive a medical degree in the United States. We all walk with you and stand on your shoulders.

Mostly, this book is for my children. Their unconditional love has helped me to climb the mountain of purgatory. They are the Beatrice to my Virgil and have guided me through what I thought was an endless journey. Purgatory can be beautiful; it's a place to start toward the discovery of how strong you are and to explore what you are going to stand up for in life.

Stand and Deliver -
A life worth fighting for

It's the age-old saying that we all love to hate; the grass is always greener on the other side.

You could be a hair-stylist who dreams of being a mechanic, or an IT guy who would love to become a carpenter.

Whatever your pipedream – we've all been there with our fantasies.

But what about if you had your career 'calling', but the odds started stacking against you?

For Kellie Stecher M.D – this was a reality. Her life was far from easy to begin with.

In a dysfunctional home with a narcissistic mother, Kellie fantasised about her 'real family', something that didn't exist – to come and find her and take her away. But that day never came – and she had to grow up a fighter, knocking back the insults as they came – mainly from her manipulative mom.

Kellie quite literally climbed her way through academia and the other uncertainties that life threw at her. Whilst becoming a mom-of-two in the process herself.

Now post-pandemic, Kellie exclusively lifts the lid on life as a female OBGYN during Covid, day-to-day medical misogyny, why doctors' depression is sky high – and what she wants to do to change it.

Her dynamic book 'Delivering' is jam-packed with the

stuff that medics never say, the opinions that are never voiced — and the inspiration for little girls, wherever they are, to get out there and make a change.

Reconciliation

Reconciliation, for those who don't know, is one of the seven sacraments of Catholicism. It is the sacrament of penance. We confess our sins, or what we perceive to be sins, to a priest and they give us advice as to how to improve, and forgive us our sins. This is for people to be absolved of their sins after baptism. This is so we can walk more closely to the Divine, as we come to understand it.

We go through this sacrament in fifth grade. Often, it's done with some pomp and circumstance. I know; I was made to go to a religious education camp. During the camp, we sang and had conversations about life and expectations. We were told how to live a more virtuous life. It was hard for me to get behind all of the religious fanfare. After all, I was baptized Methodist, despite my grandfather being a Lutheran Minister. This seems to have been in part because of some marital discord between my parents. My grandfather, whom I have always admired, baptized my other siblings and cousins.

He was one of the true heroes I had growing up. Even my mother, who didn't like many people, seemed to admire him. We were raised in the Lutheran faith until around fifth grade. At that time my father was traveling a great deal to Europe for work. My mother, in her all-knowing wisdom, took us to a Catholic church service and talked to a nun about converting us to Catholicism. We were then converted and re-baptized in another faith. I didn't really know how to feel about this dramatic departure of normal life.

When I took the sacrament of first reconciliation, we had classes and needed to pick a mentor dedicated to this religious process. I couldn't comprehend the magnitude of religion at that time. I recited exactly what I thought the leaders wanted to hear. I wasn't a dumb kid; I could certainly tell people what they wanted to hear. After all, I had practice doing that almost every day for my entire life.

I really wanted to believe in some sort of religion. I wanted to believe there was a power greater than us that would help us when we fell from grace. I wanted to be religious, spiritual, and believe everything, because if religion is real, if heaven and hell are real, there will be justice for people who do bad things, and people who work hard and help others just might be rewarded in heaven. I wanted to feel like I belonged in some way to something bigger than myself. I wanted to think there was a higher purpose than just me and my mundane existence in the world.

The last time I saw my grandfather alive, I was actually studying for a religious education class. I was sitting on my bed in the room I shared with my sister. I hated sharing a room at the time; however, I long for the days I could yell next to me and have her answer in the dark. She is one of the other main characters in my life. She has evolved to be one of my true soul mates on earth.

I was laying on my twin bed, facing the door, holding a paper with the Ten Commandments on it. I was getting frustrated about needing to study for a test on religion. I would rather be doing anything other than studying. I also felt embarrassed that my grandfather was in my house and I was studying for a Catholic test. He walked into my room because he knew I was struggling with life. He sat quietly next to me on the bed. He smiled and looked at me. His eyes were kind and calm. His smile was contagious. His hugs brought you life. He asked what the issue was. I explained that I was frustrated when I didn't get something right away. He chuckled and said, 'You have to do the things you don't want to do so you can do the things you want to do. Nothing in life comes easy, kid. You have to take one moment and one line at a time.' He kissed my forehead, hugged me goodbye, and that was the last moment we had together on this earth.

Come to think of it, I haven't been to a reconciliation in more than twenty years. With that I will start my confessions. Forgive me Father for I have sinned…

Kids and Stitches

It has been said that children pay for the sins of their parents. I think that statement can carry some legitimate truth. Nonetheless, growing up in rural Wisconsin had its perks; we were essentially feral children. We would leave in the morning and come home at dusk. As kids, we were never made to fear for our safety. We were never really worried about being kidnapped . In part, that's because the three of us were left alone on a consistent basis and watched out for one another. I remember I learned how to cook breakfast food for my siblings so we didn't just eat cereal and pizza for every meal.

One morning, during the summer before sixth grade, I was trying to cook eggs. The pan we had was broken; one of the legs was wobbly. I put the first two eggs in the pan and it fell off the edge of the counter. I reflexively caught the pan. I immediately regretted that move. I ran my hands under cold water as they both swelled and blistered immediately. Each finger had its own individual white neural-tissue-looking pad. My sister called my father at work, but we didn't have the luxury or the means for him to rush home, take time off work, and take me to the doctor. He said, 'Well, keep putting cold water on it. It will get better.' So, I dug through the cabinet, found some Neosporin, and went on with my day.

We had one car for the family used primarily to get my

father to his place of work. We would wave out the window every morning when he was departing, and the days seemed all very much the same. It was my mother, sister and I hanging out at home. One morning I decided I wanted to watch Sesame Street; even at three I was fairly independent. The large, heavy, rigid television set was on a turn table. I spun the TV toward the couch, and in that moment the ash tray on top of the entertainment center crashed down onto the top of the television. My face was washed with a spray of small glass shards. When I heard the noise, I instinctually covered me eyes. I looked up when the noise stopped. My mother, Terri, was feeding Kristen in the kitchen. I turned my face to her slowly because I could feel the burning pain on my cheeks and forehead. It felt heavy, like I was unable to move. I said, 'Mom, I think I have a hole in my face.' I was, in fact, able to palpate my cheek with my tongue and find a gap that I could slide my tongue through. I screamed, 'Look mom, I can get my tongue in my cheek.'

She calmly set my sister down and called for my father to come home. She told my dad to hurry up and get to the house now. In hindsight, I realize she didn't want me to freak out, cry, or rub my face or eyes. I was sitting in a pool of glass, fragments of wood, and blood.

When we checked into the emergency room, I was immediately seen. A young male doctor and two nurses held down my chest and arms. Dad, who has always had an inability to deal with blood or anything borderline gross, held down my legs and looked off to the wall behind him. He positioned his body away from mine, and in that moment, I felt more alone as they cleansed my skin and started pulling out the slivers of glass. I heard rumblings of calling a plastic surgeon because it was my face. But it was bleeding and specialists would have cost more money.

The two nurses, the doctor, and my dad continued to hold me down because when the stitches started, that's when the real pain happened. My face had to be closed in a couple layers. I felt each stitch searing into my cheek. I could feel the entire length of the suture as it was pulled through the muscle and skin. When it was done, I was left with a bright red scar that had the appearance of a lightning bolt.

No family is without accidents. As a mom, I definitely have learned you can't predict or control every catastrophic event. My daughter, as my dad points out, is a mini-me. She has all my very best qualities and all my very worst. As an adult, I was in clinic and received an SOS call from my husband that Addie, age three, had gashed her head open at gymnastics. I didn't hesitate to say, 'Yes, take her to the ER; I'll meet you there.' I never thought, wow, could this set me back financially. The reason: we have insurance, and despite the extremely large deductible, I am not afraid to take my kids to the doctor when they need something. In fact, I have come to terms with the reality that in current day, 2020, I will always meet my family deductible on an annual basis. When I arrived in the ER, at the hospital where I worked, I was comforted by the familiarity of the place and so was Addie, as she had been there to visit me. Whenever we drive by, she proudly proclaims that I work at the hospital and I deliver babies.

My son, husband, amazing sister, and I all sat bedside. My

sister sang to her and read books. I sat looking at her perfect little face and holding her hands. I wasn't going to turn away from her. I wanted her to know I was in the moment with her. One of my professional colleagues came in and set up numbing medication on her forehead which was to make her more comfortable. There was enough tension on the wound that it needed to be cleaned out and stitched back together. She didn't cry; she had adequate pain control. She held my hands, mostly because she was scared and not because she was in pain. She didn't need staff to hold her down. She had her family surrounding her for comfort. When we went home she played in the yard with her brother.

Growth and Grit

G rowing up, I always had to be perfect; I wanted to be the best athlete and win the academic awards. I was so critically hard on myself when I made any small error. Starting at a young age, my sister, brother, and I were left alone during the summers. My mother often had previous engagements and my father was working so that we could live.

I was an outsider in my own family. The only times I felt valued or appreciated were when I was given some sort of external validation. Then I appeared on my mother's radar in a positive way, so that's what I did; I worked endlessly. I never started a project I didn't finish. I made sure my siblings were safe and I supported them in their endeavors. I vowed never to break a promise to someone I cared about.

When I was eight, my sister was six, and my brother was four, we had been told we could go to a baseball camp. It was affiliated with the minor league baseball team we all loved. My dad got tickets frequently from his work since they were a sponsor. We would go to games and for a moment, I felt like I could do anything. When the day for the camp came, Dad had to be at work early and my mother had checked out. I dug through the couches, my dad's dresser, the coin containers. I was able to collect about $10, called a cab, and got us to the baseball camp. I wasn't going to let myself or my siblings down. When the camp was done, I called my dad from a pay phone and told him where we were. For many years, he just assumed it was planned and my mother must have dropped us off. That was the first time I knew I could stand alone to get something done for people that mattered to me.

My dad and I, unfortunately, had a particularly negative relationship during my childhood. I later came to realize that I was my mother's scapegoat. She often lied to him, blaming me or making me into the villain of her story. I will never forget the first time she kicked me out of the house. I was in fifth grade, sitting on the arm of the couch in our living room. My brother and I were arguing. In that moment, she didn't care what happened, how it came to be, or even think about my well-being. She reached across and smacked my face as hard as she could and I fell backward onto the couch. I was in shock. I didn't know what to say or how to respond. She screamed at me in a way I never thought I would witness a mother speaking to a child.

'Get out of my house you fat fucking cow.'

When I didn't immediately leap off the couch, she screamed it again, this time adding 'ugly' into the tirade. I went out the front door, slamming it closed. The light fixture above the door flew off and cracked on the ground. I took my bike and rode to my elementary school. I rode as quickly as I could as if trying to get to some higher ground of safety.

I sat at a solitary picnic table wondering when my real family would come get me. After all, this wasn't the first time she had called me fat, ugly, lazy and worthless. She'd even told me I was a mistake, or said that she didn't want me. Something in my child's mind died that day. Any love and trust that I had for her had completely vanished.

My mother told my dad how horrible I had been to her, that I was a spoiled brat. He had to do something about me. That was the key. My dad believed what my mother said. My siblings never knew what had been done until I left the house and similar things were done to them. My dad, in the last couple of years, finally realized what happened. He realized he had been overly aggressive and angry toward me, often for no reason at all. I never talked to him about it. I never thought he would listen or believe me. Instead, I shut down a huge part of myself, and learned to hate everything I was.

Every time my parents would speak to me in anger, a little voice in my head would counter it. I would tell myself I would never be like that and I would never say those things to my children. That voice started when I was four years old. I was loading the dishwasher, which now is somewhat hilarious to me as my five-year-old has never done that. My mother told me I was lazy and compared me to her sisters. I looked her square in the eyes and told her she could never hope to see her grandchildren. I didn't see a way out of this situation.

I had no money of my own and they had no money to give. I often thought I was better off dead than with these people. I would dream of my real parents coming to find me, the ones that wanted me and loved me and would support me through whatever I wanted to do and whoever I ended up being.

For a long time, we couldn't afford a basketball hoop, so I would pick areas on the driveway that were cracked or specific scuff marks on the garage door and try to hit those marks with my basketball. I would say, 'Okay, if I make this basket, win this award, get the best grade, my real family would come get me.' Unfortunately, that's how I lived my life. If I was the best at whatever scenario, got the most recognition, won the most points, then either my real family would find me or my current family would leave me alone to work.

What happens to a kid who grows up living a life of defeat and self-judgment? Well, it can only go one of two ways. For me, I wanted out. I knew I never wanted to have a family or raise children if I couldn't afford to support them. I saw my parents constant financial throw-down arguments. I knew I wanted to be as far removed from my mother's influence as possible. When I left home, I didn't look back. My sister had no idea how dysfunctional the relationship was until I left home.

One of the proudest moments of my life came at a softball game where my parents were not present, of course. My teams always became more like my family because it was the only place where I felt I belonged. In that game, I became the first girl to hit an out-of-the-park home-run, I also hit a triple and double. My teammate's dad, who was an amazing role model, well-known in the area, and had put together a celebrity team to play our minor league team, brought me my home-run ball.

He pulled out a Bolton Bombers softball from his car and wrote the date on the ball and what I had accomplished. For a kid who wasn't shown any affection by her parents, this was hugely impactful. It showed me someone saw me, valued me, and cared. Mr Slye will probably never know how important that moment was for me and that scribbled-on softball that sits on my bookshelf.

My mother Terri became a state representative when I was in high school. She lived most of her time in Madison while my dad was at home working. When you run for local government your family becomes somewhat popular in the local community. We had countless events to attend and people that were in and out of our house on a regular basis, and we had interacted with all types of people, often introducing them to others. Unfortunately, campaigns don't change behavior or hide who we really are from each other.

Our family was always recruited to do her campaigning. We made calls, mapped out constituents, put up signs, went door to door. We did it with smiles and without a thank you. We did this so we could survive without being picked apart. My sister had the great fortune of being our mother's campaign manager when she ran for a national seat. My sister ran her butt off catering to mother's every need. At one point trying to balance high school, getting into college, and running a campaign. The thanks she got came in a fit of anger when she was told, 'You're not good enough to be my wait staff.'

We have very few family photos documenting our lives. Before the last campaign she had prior to my parent's divorce, the campaign manager questioned why we didn't have an updated family photo. They planned a photography session, so there would be an image showing us as the perfect family we portrayed to the world. Terri had bought a couple of board games at Target that sat on a bookshelf. During the photography session, the individual with the camera wanted to see us in our 'natural state.' What was our natural state? Was it the fact that my mother hated us ninety-nine percent of the time, or that we were props at her disposal?

She ripped off the plastic on the board game and the five of us huddled around in silence. We took the pieces out of the plastic bags and placed them around the board. 'The pieces can't be that close together; that looks fake.' I remember the photographer making that single comment. That line played in my head because it was true. Every part of my life was fake. I held my piece and looked at my family. I realized I didn't want to play this game anymore. I wasn't going to be this blue game piece that could get moved around on a whim. I wasn't going to have people lie about me and patronize me any longer. I was done with the game.

Body Betrayal

ll my life I felt like the ugly duckling. This had led to a constellation of odd relationships created to give me some sort of positive feedback and reassurance. In some ways, I believed my body was just a functional vessel. However, I was tall: there's a positive I tried to focus on. I loved basketball, so this was perfect. I could totally get behind the WNBA or Rowing.

Growing up, constantly hearing the feedback that I was fat or ugly was something that I fought on a daily basis. My mother didn't need to continue saying these things because, after a few years, I took the mantle up for her. I avoided mirrors and rarely interacted with people of the opposite sex. I never felt good enough or even thought someone would be attracted to me.

I was always the tallest person in class photos, sometimes to an awkward and disproportionately traumatizing level. I had breasts first. My mother was clearly in denial until one of her friends commented that I needed to start wearing bras

I was a tomboy. Every recess, I would play tackle football with the boys in the back fields of the elementary school, right where the grass met the farm fields. Yes, my Amazonian self was significantly bigger than the majority of the kids who played. One fall day, rain was starting to come in. The fields were getting wet, the grass was slippery, and the game was getting more frustrating to play. I ran deep in the field. I was wide open and signaled to the quarter back. When it was one of my friends at QB, I could get the ball. We knew each other; we played sports in the street in front of where I lived. In this moment he threw the ball to a boy that was less equipped and smaller, and he fumbled it. I couldn't believe what happened. It was the first time I recognized being discriminated against because I was a girl. The little boy that was covering me started laughing because we had lost. I yelled to the QB, 'What happened? I was wide?!? We would have won!'

The little boy covering me, screamed, 'Yeah, you're wide!' That little boy, Aaron, was a runt. He was petite, un-athletic, unapologetic, and treated people poorly. However, in that moment, I gave him all my power. See, the disparaging voice shifted from my mom to me, to the little boys that I played with on the fields. Before this moment, I was doing a fine job telling myself how horrible I was. I honestly didn't know how to process someone taking over that role.

My life became a constant array of awkward moments associated with my height and build and people thinking I was older than I was. When people see your physical person and make judgements and decisions in how to treat you from there on out, it's powerful and harmful when you're a kid. I just wanted to belong. I wanted to fit in, not stick out, to blend in with the crowd.

In fifth grade, by some miracle, I had found another tall girl to have as a friend. I had a brood of lovely athletic boys I hung out with. I started seeing my stature as a blessing and not a curse. I became more social, much to the chagrin of my teachers. I was in class at Houdini Elementary School in Appleton. I had somehow found the nerve to have a modicum of self-confidence. I was in sports. I could walk to and from school. I had my group of friends. I was extremely strong academically and hoped that would bolster my relationships at home.

One day I was sitting next to one of my boy friends in class. I was done early with the math work and was bored and there weren't other people done to talk with. I turned to him and asked what was going on. He was struggling and didn't understand a component of the problem. I started telling him what I did. The teacher heard the conversation, and yelled out, 'If you think you can teach the class better than me, then by all means come up here.'

I agreed to take on the challenge, 'Ok, sounds good to me.' I made the walk to the chalkboard. I pulled open a book and wrote out the math problem I was helping Bryan with. I explained it, showed my work, and before I could sit down, she called me into the hallway.

We were ten feet from the room. We were near the stairwell down to the library, and I remember staring down the steps wishing I could run. She looked at me and began to give me her opinion.

'You think you can back talk to me in class?'

'I'm sorry I was just trying to help him with the problem. He wasn't understanding.'

'So, you think you can do the job better than I can? You are not going anywhere in life with that attitude. You are going nowhere!'

Well again, to someone who is barely holding themselves together and has limited self-confidence, this annihilated any remnant that was on my radar. I went from being proud that I could help a classmate to feeling like the worthless girl my mother always said I was.

However, if there is one thing I knew, it was how enraged my mother became when something reflected poorly on her. I told her the story and she of course did what I knew she would. She flew into that school and set everyone straight. My mother couldn't believe that a teacher would talk to a child my age like she did. The principal brought up that I looked much more adult than I really was, as if that was an excuse. The big problem was that the emotional damage was done.

My hatred toward my body was constant at that point. At age ten, I wasn't given candy by a neighbor because I was too old and told I needed to let kids enjoy Halloween. That was the last time I went trick-or-treating. In sixth grade, my grandfather died and at the visitation, I was standing next to my sister and brother, people thought I was my mother. They kept talking to me about my looks, how youthful I appeared. 'That's because I am in sixth grade, Sir.' Being mistaken for my mother was a bridge too far for me.

As I grew up, I started having the luxury of blending in more. I slouched down to make myself smaller in an effort to be non-intimidating. The adult me is so disappointed that no one had an intervention with teenage me. I didn't realize that you shouldn't shrink yourself to make others more comfortable. The most amazing people don't fit in in this world. The world changers aren't blending into their surroundings.

I got to the point where I was 100 percent convinced no boy would ever like me for me. I would tell myself that I was smart, I cared about people, I worked hard, but you know no teenage boy likes those things. They're interested in being popular and having a perfect image. Sadly, the heart wants what it wants and - despite me knowing I wasn't good enough for different suitors, I still wanted to go for it.

I had a classmate who would talk to me periodically. He seemed sweet and genuine. He also wasn't perfect by any stretch of the imagination. (Of course we can talk about how men who are not nearly perfect think their wives, girlfriends, women who just gave birth to their children need to be perfect?)

I will never understand how this disconnect started. You see amazing attractive women with below average looking guys all the time because he's a good guy, he treats her well. The average and below average looking women... well, you aren't likely to win a prince charming over.

Nevertheless, I thought this young boy was great, not because of how he looked, but how he treated other people. I thought he was an awesome athlete. He was smart and did well in school. When I told him I liked him, it was by way of asking him to a school dance where girls are supposed to ask guys. Of course, I made this call while sitting in the middle of my bedroom, on a phone with a long cord that I managed to tangle around my leg during a fit of nerves. During the call, my sister was staring blankly at me, full of anxiety, like she was going through this herself. My dad happened to pick up the phone while I was trying to pretend to be a flirty and desirable girl. I just remember getting the word, 'dance,' out of my mouth, and I heard my dad dialing, and his deep booming voice, 'Hello, hello, someone there.'

'Nope, no one is here.' I responded, and honestly in that moment of teenage panic, I wanted to be no one.

After the call ended, I was fully convinced I would be single forever. He seemed nice on the phone, and I shrugged it off. Low and behold it was quite comical to him that I thought this football player would ever go for the tall basketball playing girl. I would love to say this is the first, and last time someone made a public joke out of my feelings, but sadly that is not the case.

I was sad, not in a heart-broken way, but because I had put myself out there and this is what I got in return. So, I devised a plan. We had just gotten AOL, America Online, dial-up internet. I knew what this young man's screen name was on AOL. I made up a username to talk to him. I was convinced I was going to be like Cyrano de Bergerac and would win his love by showing him who I was on the inside. Now, the genius here is that I was catfishing before catfishing was a thing. After school I would run home, hop on the computer and we would talk, sometimes for hours. He thought I was a teenager his age, from a neighboring school. I sent him poetry on love, which he claimed to enjoy. He decided he loved me and wanted to meet. He said things like 'it was meant to be' and 'we are meant to be together.' Then, I told him who I was... Silence in any situation can be painful. But, in matters of the heart it can feel deadly. To him, I was perfect, I was a soul mate, I was everything he wanted... Until he knew what I looked like.

I spent the rest of my high school years focused on me and surviving to get out of my house and moving to college. I was solely dedicated to being successful in whatever I wanted to do. I had many friends from grades above me, mostly because I was in a higher band level than many my age. I was that girl, the alto saxophone playing, jazz band participating in, poetry journal writing, rowing kind of girl. Mostly I was trying to find a home base, somewhere I could be myself and be accepted and accomplish what I wanted to achieve.

My senior year I went to a party. This party was college-like and had kegs of beer. I personally hated beer, and always will. It probably stems from my associations with the beverage from the first time I tried it when my dad let me have a sip. I almost vomited right then and there. I could taste the mix of cigarettes and alcohol and my six-year-old self wasn't having it. As I got older, the taste of beer made me regret kisses that I had with young and old men after drinking.

I left the party and laid out on the front lawn looking up at the stars. I spent so much of my life hoping for the next phase to come. In this moment I was attempting to just exist in the world, as a human being. Since I had given up on boys, I had no desire to stay in an over-crowded room. In that moment Greg showed up. He was significantly older than I was; he had a job, he appeared to be holding it together, and, for some strange reason, he seemed to be interested in me. He lay down next to me in the grass. I was immediately skeptical.

'Do I know you?'

'No, but you're beautiful and seem nice and I thought you could use the company.'

Every bit of that sentence was highly suspect. I, after all, couldn't be perceived by anyone to be beautiful. I almost choked on laughter when he continued to compliment me. It was funny and then it was a dream. Maybe I wouldn't die old and alone with my twenty dogs, because I am not a cat person. He walked me to his car because he wanted to get my number. We had to do it the old-fashioned way with a pen and paper. He grabbed me and kissed me. It was the first time I ever had a tongue in my mouth that wasn't my own. I'm fairly certain I was paralyzed in shock and unable to participate. I just remember the taste of sour beer.

Always Wear Spanx

Well, when he called, I answered. Actually, my dad, who seemed to be the guardian of the phone, answered and then allowed me to speak. We set up a date. He was going to pick me up and we were going to go to dinner of some sort. I wore a skirt; it was too warm to wear nylons. However, any self-conscious girl knows you don't leave home without Spanx.

I did a quick look in the mirror. As I sat staring at my reflection, I really didn't understand why I was going on this date. After all, I barely knew him, and his biggest ambition was to never leave the small town we grew up in. But he seemed to like me, and that was the basis of a compelling argument.

I ran out the door as soon as the car pulled up. As we were driving, he told me he needed to pick up a couple remaining things from his apartment. He was moving out and thought there was one box that needed to be collected. He promised it would only take a second or two. When we got to the apartment complex I should have waited in the car. I should have gotten out and called someone to pick me up. However, as a seventeen-year-old girl on a date with a much older guy who is strong and confident, there isn't a lot of room for error. I also didn't even think I had anyone I could depend on coming to get me.

We walked up the stairs to the apartment that was basically

empty. Some cleaning supplies on the kitchen counter. It was dusk outside. Inside there were no lamps and nothing to turn on to light the living room where I was standing. He started walking away and then turned back and pushed me against the wall. He kissed me so aggressively I couldn't breathe. It was like I was frozen. I didn't know what to do or what to say.

I had no one who could come get me. This was a time before cell phones. I was fairly confident that if I died, it would be a very long time before someone found me. When he knocked me into the wall, I hit my head fairly hard. I felt wet on the back of my head and something ran down my neck. I remembered that we were in an apartment complex and I hit my fist against the wall between the other apartment and the one we were in.

The next thing I remember I had slid down the wall and he was sitting on my chest. I hit the wall again as hard as I could. He was sitting in a way that I was struggling to get air to fill my lungs. He grabbed my face, and I tried to look away. I had always had a hard time making eye contact with men, mostly because I was afraid of the relationships I had had in the past. He ripped my skirt up and, in that moment, I was so thankful for the tight, hot, sweaty Spanx that were on my body.

He asked, 'What the fuck is this? Can you even get out of these?'

He reached down and stuck his fingers in my vagina and asked, 'why are you so tight?'

'I'm a virgin,' I said.

Now, the adult me is horrified and traumatized that that came out of my mouth. Some men, especially men who are trying to force you to do something, do feel like being a virgin is a turn on. And that's something I quickly realized with how he responded to the statement.

I didn't know what else to say. I was trying to hit the wall, get up, get out from under him, breathe, all of it. He was struggling to get my Spanx off and I was struggling to make enough noise that someone would find my body before it decayed.

I finally found my voice, I started screaming. I told him, 'I'm seventeen! If you rape me, it isn't just rape, it's statutory rape. I'm seventeen! The neighbors saw us come in.'

With that he got off my chest. My Spanx mostly intact, but I left bruised and battered.

When I walked through the door, I couldn't look at anyone. My parents were in the living room and they didn't notice the gash on the back of my head and neck from the metal door stop I hit when I was pushed to the floor. The cut on my scalp from the nail that was in the wall that had once held a pleasant photograph of this man. I went to my bed, still in my Spanx, and pulled the covers over my body. I laid there in a cocoon. I said nothing, I did nothing. I didn't move for twelve hours.

In an effort to belong and feel worthy of love, I put myself in a situation where I could have died. I could have been raped. I could be pregnant. All because I just wanted someone to love me or want me. I wanted someone to see me. Honestly, there were many times after that that I wished he would have just sat for a minute longer on my neck or hit my head harder. Because dealing with the fall out of some of these things has left more emotional scars then physical.

This moment, a period of ninety minutes that I experienced as a teenager, changed the way I talk to people. Teenagers need to be educated on how to best protect themselves. As horrible as it is to say, we as women, need to be smart to survive these things. I wish I would have had a person that I could have called anytime, anywhere, that would have dropped everything to come get me. Knowing I had that, in that moment, may have saved that entire situation. We need to change the conversation around sex and sexual violence with women and teenagers. We need to have open dialogue so they aren't paralyzed in these moments and know they are strong and can fight and deserve to survive.

Online Dating Before Online Dating Existed

When I was in my pre-teens and early teen years, Bill Clinton was president. I was sitting in the living room next to my father, watching the televised speeches responding to Monica Lewinsky. I immediately knew he was lying, and I was so disgusted by this man in power. When you're that age, you feel like you know everything. You have this strong moral compass, and you are outraged for all injustices. Truth be told, I think I have actually gravitated more toward who I was then as of recent years. I wanted a fight; I was looking for someone to do verbal battle with.

I went to the computer and waited the 100 minutes before the dial up internet connected to AOL. Once I got logged on, I opened the search for people profiles area. At that time, you could look for phrases or words that were in people's online AOL profiles. Additionally, you could tell who was active because there was a green dot next to their screen name. I typed in the phrase, 'I love Bill Clinton.' Well, there happened to be several individuals with that very phrase logged onto the computer, at that very moment. I happened to pick the first one alphabetically and decided to message him.

'What is wrong with you? He clearly is abusing his power and making up lies about an intern!'

'Well, hello, I'm Joe...'

And the rest is history… really, this is who I ended up marrying.

Every time I logged on to do schoolwork he would message me and essentially try to start a debate. He took great pride in fighting with me. I could definitely hold my own. Of course, I lied and told him my name was Katie, I was blonde, short, petite, from Minnesota and not Wisconsin. I had no idea if he was a serial killer.

After years of banter, we became sort of pen pals. He went away to school at University of Maryland and stayed there in the summers to do internships. He ended up being lonely at times, and I became a random voice in the void of life. Five years of talking quickly passed and he asked me if I thought we should meet. I immediately hated the idea. First of all, I'm not some cute petite kid named Katie, and I had no proof he wasn't going to serial kill me. I said I hated the idea. I didn't even know if he was who he said he was since, clearly, I knew I wasn't divulging my true identity.

He sent me a care package. In the package was a cluster of pictures, a letter, a teddy bear that had a shirt, 'Someone at University of Maryland Loves Me.' That threw me off my game. I was really not going to ever meet him. I couldn't imagine a scenario in which meeting him would lead to any positive outcome for either one of us.

We had a couple months of negotiation about meeting. During this time, I slowly came forward with details of simple things, like that I was actually an Amazonian woman. We coordinated a meeting over his Christmas break. My university started in early January and he had almost the entire month free, so in January 2002 he came to visit me. I point that out so you might have a historical context for the outfit I am about to describe. He rolled up in a giant station wagon, which he called 'The Beast.' It was his parents' car, which was essentially indestructible because both he and his brother learned to drive in it. He was wearing pleated jeans, a Muppets t-shirt, and a black leather jacket. All my girlfriends from the dorm were there to investigate; we're talking easily twenty sets of eyeballs to make sure I wasn't the first murdered coed from St. Mary's.

After they all suitably vetted him and deemed him a non-threat to my safety, we were allowed to go on a date. Where did he take me? Well, we went down the road to McDonald's. Even for a freshman in college, this seemed less than ideal and certainly not any sliver of romantic flavor. He asked what I wanted and I got a soda. We sat in a booth and he decided to try to sit next to me. I slid out the other side and sat across from him.

'I don't share sides of the booth with anyone. Unless there are another two people with us, I get my own side.'

We made it through the date and went for a walk. It was very odd being with him in real time. For our grand second date, he decided we were going to go to my college cafeteria, and I was fortunate enough to buy. This meant I didn't get one of my dinners or lunches for the rest of the week.

After the date was done, I had decided we weren't a love match. He didn't seem to be making any effort; I was just there. He didn't even get the door for me and never made any plans. He also ate like he was in prison, holding his fork like a baton. He said his goodbyes and I did the super mature thing any eighteen-year-old would do; I decided to break up with him over email. I sent him a letter that I just wasn't feeling the connection and thought we were better off not pursuing a romantic relationship.

He read the email when he got home and tried calling several times. Each time my roommate answered and came up with another story. My best friend Megan, said, 'Yeah definitely dump him, no effort now means no effort later.' He then wrote me a love letter. The letter was actually really beautiful. In it he told me he loved me, and he couldn't imagine his life without me since I had been in his life for five years before this. If I gave him another chance, he would treat me how I needed to be treated. Well, that did it. We got married July 1, 2006 and we have two beautiful kids.

Empaths Unite!

The things I have told myself my entire life is I am smart, I can do this, and someone will love me for my brain. Also, that I have a good personality; when they are older, men will just fall in love with my sense of humor.

However, some of us have an almost pathological need to win someone over. Then, we act surprised when they throw us under the bus, just like everyone warned us they would. For this, I blame science. The data shows, in fact, that male abusers and those that would perpetrate toxic relationships often go for strong, confident, and successful women. Successful women tend to be more conscientious, perfectionistic, detail oriented, and have higher emotional intelligence and empathy. This tends to create the perfect storm for a successful empath to form a friendship or relationship with someone who will take advantage of all his or her personality traits.

Empaths are individuals who have increased sensitivity to those around them and feel the pain of others more acutely than the average person. These individuals often need to be told that the fight isn't their battle because they take on other people's problems as their own. They're sensitive to the vibe in a room or the emotions of people around them.

Romantic relationships can often lead these people to lose sight of themselves and focus on making a partner happy. An empath absorbs an intimate partner's energy, and when his or her mood is off it can significantly affect the empath's mood. This is a good reason why many should not date co-workers or have any sort of intimate relationship with them.

Often, empaths want others to like them. They want to make people happy and work on the family or work culture. These people don't understand why leaders can't put their staff or other people first because it feels innate to them. Also, they have a strong need for justice. Unfortunately, these qualities feed toxic individuals because the latter are aware that these people want positive reinforcement from the relationship. They have now been given the road map to weaponize all the traits that everyone else had loved about empaths.

In medical school, there is a strong focus on creating physicians who are empathetic. In healthcare these individuals can thrive. However, it's important they are not taken advantage of. As an empath myself, I can see the slippery slope of needing to help others at all cost, and always trying to make people happy. The destructive part is really only done to yourself. In any field you pursue it's important to create healthy boundaries and not lose sight of who you are.

Until recently, I completely identified with my job as a physician. Many people lose themselves to their work. However, I felt that without my job I was nothing. I think my personality significantly played a role in my self-identification with work. It becomes a compulsive need to be present, do everything you can, not let someone else down. I'm hoping this discussion will help someone out there like me be able to separate work from life and maybe even avoid some misguided relationships. Healthcare can be great for these personalities.

You can use all your layers to relate to people; just don't get used by the wrong leaders and colleagues.

Stay in the Boat

I have always been competitive to the largest degree possible. When I was in junior high school, I was getting almost 100 percent in my history class. Our teacher handed out extra credit work and, of course, I had to do the work. To memorize the Gettysburg Address. I wanted to be the student who memorized it in the shortest amount of time and was able to recite it the fastest and clearest in class. I can still remember the vast majority of the address. Now, why on earth did I need to do this? My 'A' looked the same as someone who had a 93 percent. I realized I didn't want it unless I could be the best at it. I was officially an all-or-nothing person; my need to be perfect was essentially a way of being self-destructive. It was my way to minimize anything I did if it wasn't perfection.

In High School, I got recruited for the crew, the tall person's sport. There was more focus on Title IV and women's athletics at that time. Rowing was one of the sports that colleges were investing in, in terms of scholarships, time, equipment and money.

Rowing was an escape from reality for me. I would wake up around 4:30 a.m. for the 5:00 practice. My brother was pre-pubescent at the time, so he weighed maybe eighty pounds. This made him the perfect coxswain. Coxswains sit at the head of the boat and steer. Since they are essentially dead weight, you want them to be as light as possible. My poor sister got roped into practice as well. Usually, we rowed with a boat of four, sweeps rowing. We would get to the boathouse, open up the garage doors, pick up the boat and place it on our shoulders to walk out to the dock. There was nothing better than getting the boat out as the sun was rising. There was something about the water, the calm, and the beginning of a new day. When our boat was moving and we were all swinging together, it felt like our team could do anything. The sound of the oars cutting into the water, pulling the weight, and lifting up like feathers was enough to warm my heart.

Our boat of four was training for a 'sprints' race that was 2,000 meters. We had about a week left of practice before the race. Despite the fact that it looked like the sky was going to open up and downpour, we decided to take the boat out on the water. We were well down the Fox river in full practice mode when the storm came. We turned the boat around and raced back to the docks. The entire time our boat was taking in water. Our coach kept screaming at us from the little fishing boat next to us to watch our technique. We couldn't lose the boat in the water, and we couldn't unstrap our feet or we wouldn't be able to keep rowing. All four of us kept our feet laced into the boat and continued to row just as we had. At one point the people on the dock said it looked like we were sitting directly on the water. The entire boat had gone under and the only sign it was there was the four of us trying to move against the storm. Once we got to the dock, we all ran and got buckets and bailed out the boat so we could lift it up and out of the river.

I was energized by our ability to work through this and get our training in. However, one of the girls quit shortly after. All-or-nothing people need to realize that most people aren't all-or-nothing. Most people don't want to row through life's storms. The world needs people who are going to stay strapped in at all costs. We only make progress because people are willing to pull the weight of the oars.

The Twin Towers

I was a freshman living in Benilde Hall and finally was starting to live the life I wanted. I was working to build my new friendships and start first semester off right. I had just opened the door to my dorm room to get into the hallway when I saw my friend Kelly moving rapidly toward me.

'Did you hear? Did you hear what's going on?'

Of course not, I was hustling to get to class. My face clearly answered her question.

'Turn on the TV Kell; it's all over the news. There has been some sort of accident in New York.'

I remember I knocked on my best friend Megan's door; she was going to walk to class with me. We turned on the TV and watched the second crash. We watched them replay the crashes over and over. We didn't know what happened. We didn't know how this would change our lives. It seemed to me if there were two crashes, it couldn't have just been an accident. We then heard about Washington, the Pentagon, the other planes, and all the other events unfolding across the country. My friend, who became my husband, was living near DC at the time. Of course, I had no way of getting hold of him as neither one of us had a cell phone.

We all sat watching in silence. I don't think there was anything any one of us could have said that would have been particularly intuitive or reassuring at that time. We were a bunch of 17 and 18-year-old kids who really had no idea what this would mean for the country or the world.

On that day, September 11 2001, I decided I was going to join the military. I came from a military family. In fact, on my mother's side of the family, my sister, brother and I were the first not to be involved in some way with one of the branches. I was proud that I had a long heritage of showing up when we were needed. I thought about it; what branch would I join? Of course, it had to be the Marines. I made some calls and the next day a recruiter met me in our school library. I had initially thought, how would I recognize him? Well, of course, he came in uniform. He was poised, crisp, strong. I admired him for owning his convictions. It didn't help that my seventeen-year-old self probably would have run away with him if he asked. I filled out the paperwork. He looked at me and smiled.

'I thought you were at least eighteen. Is this your DOB?'

'Yeah, my birthday is in a couple weeks. Can I fill it out now and then have my start day be September 28th?'

'No ma'am, call in me a couple weeks if you don't change your mind. Do you know what your major is going to be?'

'Biology or chemistry, I am going pre-med.'

'Well, think about how you best want to serve your country; sometimes becoming a doctor is a better way than being on the battlefield,' the recruiter said.

My emotions flooded me. Could he secretly feel I was someone who cried at sappy movies? Did I smile too much? The events of that day colored a lot of my college career. We would be sitting in the cafeteria and the news of the ensuing conflict would be all that was broadcast. At some point it all didn't feel real. The aftershocks were, in many ways, too much for teenagers to process. However, I think it started my friends and I down the road toward servant leadership and trying to act in ways that would be virtuous and kind. Most of my college friends have spent their careers in some sort of service to the people in the communities around them.

Ready or Not

During the summer months, between my freshmen and sophomore year of college, I decided to become a certified nursing assistant. I did the certificate program at Fox Valley Technical College, which was down the street from where we lived. I learned how to make beds, to prepare food, and to use medical equipment. I learned how to change bed pans, give sponge baths, transfer people and lift them without hurting my back. My clinical rotations took place at the same time my grandmother was put into hospice for her oesophageal cancer.

My rotations happened to be at a nursing home. Some of the occupants had severe memory concerns; some were unable to walk, speak, hear or engage with anyone. With every patient I took care of, I saw my grandmother. I felt guilty every day being there and not with her. My second day at the assisted care facility, there was a woman who had, overnight, become incontinent. I went in to get all my patients ready to come for breakfast. I went to check in on her and she was crying. She was embarrassed, she was vulnerable, she needed me to help get her together so she could go on with her day.

I looked into her eyes and I saw my grandmother, without me there, unaware of the world around her. My mother, sister, brother and I had been with her in the hospital for her surgery. We hugged her, kissed her, talked to her. You see, that's the easy part of love. When people are fine, and you recognize them in themselves, that's easy. It takes strength to face the people you love and not be able to recognize them. It takes unconditional love and courage to walk in the door and care for someone who isn't the person you've always loved. To be there, in sickness and in health, and to be there as a loved one who would never abandon your people.

I couldn't judge the families for not visiting my patients. I couldn't fault anyone for being frustrated, angry and sad. I was not any less guilty in my family situation. The three of us kids and my mother, Terri, had walked into my grandmother's hospice room only days before this event. We were scared, we were quiet, we didn't know what to say or do. Instead of finding courage to love through the fear, we walked out. Sure, she didn't know we were there. She was unable to interact with us. However, courage should exist where love does.

That summer was my introduction to patient care. I decided in these moments I was going to lean in when things were hard. I wasn't going to run or to take the easy way out. I wasn't going to turn my back on anyone who needed my help. I was going to smile, hold hands, hug them when them needed a hug, and embrace the life we have and had. These are choices we all need to make for ourselves and how we want to show up for our loved ones. We need to ask ourselves how we want to participate in the world. We need to determine whether or not we will find strength in love or if it will break us down.

Kellie Lease Stecher, MD

Coming Out

We are all products from an intricate dance between genetics and the environment in which we live. We are born into whatever family we are, not by choice, but by luck. We look however we look because of the delicate DNA sequencing. These are all things we have no control over. We can't control what we look like, the sound of our voice, how loud our laughs are. However, I have tried to control my laugh and it is an entity on a stage all of its own. My patients always tell me they can hear me down the hall or as they walk into the clinic. That laugh is one I have earned from pure joy. My patients and my children are able to tap into the best part of me and, despite being asked to tone it down, I can't control that element of who I am.

My family was raised in a small town in northeast Wisconsin. I loved the community I grew up in. We had an excellent public educational system from which I was able to launch my career. However, the other parts of the globe did not intrude on Appleton. We weren't exposed to anyone who was different, who needed anything special, who could teach us how to be healthy well-rounded human beings. It's not my parents' fault; they both grew up in small and more rural towns than I did.

I was raised with some pretty significant biases and really an inability to even conceptualize what those biases were and how they contributed to social injustice. I am truly shocked that some of the friends I have had over the years are still my friends and loved me through my evolution into adulthood.

I had always been the square peg in the round hole. I spoke my mind and formed my own opinions. As I grew up, I would definitely speak up when I didn't agree with the actions of my parents. I fought hard to get out and move away. When I was in college, I found my stride, my people, the biology department, the amazing girls I studied with, my best friends in life, and was exposed to all the things a well-educated person should have experience with. I excelled in my classes, I volunteered, I played intra-mural-sports, and made life-long friendships.

When I was a was a sophomore, I decided to be a Resident Assistant. I became a little bit like the house mom. I was the one with the car. Although less than appealing, my little white Neon with peeling paint certainly could pick up a drunk person here and there so they didn't drive home. I was there, present, door open, ready for whatever anyone needed. Because, honestly, I wanted someone to be that person for me. I felt like if I could help someone with a broken heart, science project, edit a paper or watch a movie with, I was game.

I clearly gave off goody two shoe vibes because for Christmas one of my lovely male residents gave me a 'massager'. I opened this purple gift and was like, 'sweet, he must know I am stressed, what a great back massager'. I had it sitting, out in the open, for anyone to see, with my door always ajar. It was in fact, a vibrator. This reality didn't dawn on me until my boyfriend came to visit, and asked why the heck I had a vibrator sitting out in plain sight. Yup, that was, in-fact, how clueless I was about anything sexually related. Clearly destined to become a gynaecologist.

At this point in my life my sister and I had become really close. She was trapped at home with my parents in a sinking ship. At sixteen she would drive across the state to see me for a weekend getaway. I would not want my sixteen-year-old, with no cell phone, a marginally working car, and no credit card to drive multiple hours by herself with only a map quest print out. However, that was more normal then.

When she came to visit, we ended up playing board games and cards with a few of my residents. There was the most wonderful guy in my dorm. He became a friend because he was kind, sincere, and thoughtful. I would check in on him, and he would check in on me as well, which I have found as a sort of house mom, not really many people wanted to do. He played a game with my sister, and I just loved him so much I thought this is it, I am going to marry my sister off to this guy.

So, the next moment I had alone with him I was feeling very cheeky about the plans I had.

'Jake! What do you think of my sister? She's cute, smart, sweet.'

'Yeah, she's great.'

'What would you think if I set you up!? I think you would be so cute.'

'Kellie, she's not my type.'

'What do you mean, she's great.'

'Yeah, she's great. But, she's not my type.'

I looked at him like ok, another foolish boy I was mistaken

about. I was totally thinking he and I have a good vibe, maybe he could be my brother one day. Whatever, fine, go date an idiot girl who will cater to your every need. After a pause…

'Kellie, you can't tell anyone this.'

'Ok…'

'I haven't told anyone.'

'Ok…' Thinking maybe he's dating someone or leaving the school or whatever.

'Kellie, I am going to date men.'

I didn't skip a beat. I actually was so relieved he wasn't the fool I was making him out to be in my mind. I loved it, loved him, couldn't care less. He hadn't told his family or friends. He was afraid to because here we sat in a catholic institution. Most of our families were religious, many weren't open-minded. Many didn't understand that everyone was different and love is love.

This moment changed my thinking about love, attraction, and happiness. This moment made me feel like I could come out as who I was. Jake helped me become stronger and more confident in my own skin. As we talked, I realized a lot of his feelings about being gay, were my feelings about existing in the world. I was worried what other people thought. I was worried about how others perceived me. He helped me re-write my love for people. I was honored that he trusted me, and I was so proud of him for being able to live his truth. I couldn't say the same about myself at that time. In fact, it has taken thirty-six years for me to be able to say that with any sort of certainty and determination. And, here he was, a teenage boy, living his truth, willing to fight for true love. Willing to fearlessly love himself enough to enter into relationships that were not built on lies.

In the present Jake is married to the love of his life and they have become new fathers. I hope we can all be so lucky to find the family or soul family that will love us in our entirety and wholeness.

What do you think about when you're alone?

When I was a senior in college, the scramble to get into medical school was moving at a frantic pace. I had successfully gotten through all my MCAT prep and did fine on the test. My grades were great. I had wonderful letters of recommendation. I was proud of the application I was able to put forward and I felt odd packaging up these applications and sending them out. Each application was like a little part of my soul in a mailbox.

I only applied to a couple places in the Midwest. I knew I wanted to be in Minnesota or Wisconsin. I had spent my entire life readying myself for these moments. I already felt like I sacrificed a lot to get to the point where I was in my academic career. This, of course, was all before computerized applications, and every school had different applications, essays, and short answer portions. They required things to be notarized, packaged up, and sent. When I slid them into the postal box, I felt sick to my stomach. There was literally nothing more I could do to convince these people that I was worth a shot, or at least an interview.

I started hearing back and scheduling in-person interviews. However, Mayo sent me a thin letter, which usually only means one thing, that I have been rejected. To my surprise, they wanted to start with a phone interview as the initial screening process for an in-person interview. Word on the medical community street was that there were so many medical students who were depressed or attempted suicide they were trying to make sure they only accepted candidates that were the most mentally sound. I, being the extreme perfectionist I am, called them as soon as I made the walk across the plaza, up the four flights of stairs, to my room in Heffron hall. I scheduled the event and marked it in the planner, done.

During the application process, I was working on my senior research. Oddly enough, I was working on the effects that genistein, a phyto-estrogen (a compound that naturally occur in plants), could have on sperm samples of the Mus musculus. Basically, I was trying to see if putting mice on an estrogen-like product would affect sperm production, which potentially lead to further research or extrapolate to other animals or humans. In hindsight, knowing I was going to go into OBGYN and love taking care of patients with infertility concerns, this project made perfect sense. However, at the time, I was clearly in denial of what I was passionate about, and was still telling everyone I was going into pediatrics.

Anyone who knows me knows I am horrified of rodents. While a resident, I had a mouse problem. I was post call, walked through the door, was going to get a snack and apprehended three mice at various locations in my kitchen. After that incident, there was no way I could have slept there. I, of course, did what anyone would do; go into emergency mode, ring the bell, light the sirens, called my co-resident who saw I was in such a state of trauma that she got me into her basement so I could sleep post call.

On this day of my Mayo phone interview, I made my way to

the science building where the mice were being held. I got out the food, pulled out my concoction of phyto-estrogens to give them, opened up one of the cages, and honestly, could never have been prepared for the site I saw. I fully realize as an adult, biology major, you should not name your animals. Never under any circumstances should you do this. However, I hated the thought of handling mice and was trying to make this less traumatic for me. I gave each mouse a name. I had some mild affection toward a little chubby guy I called Gus Gus, from Cinderella. I meanwhile hated his roommate because it felt like he was always trying to attack me. So, I called him Bitey.

When I opened the cage both Bitey and Gus Gus, had perished. To make it epically worse, Bitey ate Gus Gus, well at least the front part of his body. I let out a scream like the devil had snuck up behind me and was taking me home. My advisor came down the hallway. I must have looked like a ghost. I was shaking, feeling sick, and honestly so horrified that one of the mice ate the other one. He looked at me, and very calmly told me that those things happen. You have to be prepared for the things you think you can't prepare for. He disposed of the remains for me so I didn't have to be a part of the cremation process. With that I realized I was going to be late for my very exciting phone interview and ran back to my dorm.

My dorm was old and historic, I loved the classic architecture. I sat at my desk overlooking the trees behind the building. I had the windows open. It was a beautiful day. You could hear the leaves rustling against each other. There was no place at that school more calming to me than looking out at the trees behind Heffron, and as a senior I got to do it every day from my room. The other beauty was this amazing orange and red fiery tree on the path to the science building. In the fall, I swear it was more beautiful than the burning bush. My last year I would take an extra second every day to look at the leaves before they fell.

The phone rang....

I could feel this small area in the middle of my neck just start to itch. It seemed to be getting bigger each time the phone rang. I answered, in my most professional, 'please take me, I will do a good job, and I promise to be a good physician' voice. The person on the phone explained to me the format for the interview. She wasn't going to respond verbally to my statements. She was going to ask a series of questions and write down my answers. After analysis of the responses, they would gather a pool for an in-person interview.

I have got this, I thought to myself. Trying to be my own hype man. I can totally do this. I am a catch. I work hard, I try no matter what, I think I'm smart. I had just lost like 100 pounds and was feeling more confident. I got this; I can do this.

'What's your full name?'

See already, 100% on the test, I can do this.

'Where are you from?'

'What type of music do you listen to?'

'When you are alone what do you think of?'

Hmmm. When I am alone what do I think of... like at night or day? Ok, don't sound psycho in your response. Oh man I hope Gus Gus didn't feel pain, that looked horrible. Ok, alone, uhhh, am I going to get into medical school? Am

I going to be able to pay for medical school? Is my entire life worthless up until this point if I don't get accepted? Should I really be getting married? Do I want to go to medical school? It actually sounds horrible and you're making it sound worse lady?

'I think about my family and just hope for them to be successful in whatever they do.' Hoping that sounded remotely genuine.

'Ok, I am going to say some words and you use them in a sentence or say what you associate them with... Hope.'

Oh man, I hope I graduate now that some of my mice died. I hope that I figure out what I want to do when I don't get in... Hope hope hope. There's a character Hope on one of those soap operas.

'Where there's life, there's hope.' Wait... did that just come out of my mouth. Where there is life, there is hope! Wow, I am fairly certain I plucked that from the same darn soap opera that that character exists in.

She thanked me for my time. Told me they would contact me when the final decisions were made, and with that the call ended. To not leave you in suspense, that was the last time I heard from Mayo until my residency interviews.

Helen

When you get into medical school, you're met with an incomprehensible number of new challenges. Anatomy is a first-year class and I felt like I had been mentally preparing for this class for ten years. After all, I knew I wanted to be a doctor by the time I turned four years old. Despite all my efforts, it is still the class I approached with the most trepidation. At Medical College of Wisconsin, we were given the privilege of using human cadavers on which to learn all the nuances of the human body. Many medical schools across the country have now changed to simulators, virtual anatomy lessons, and sharing a small number of cadavers for a large class.

Once we completed first year orientation, we were assigned to our anatomy groups of five to six people. These students were about to become my new best friends. Our group banded together to meet this unique set of challenges. On the first day, we all changed into scrubs to enter the lab. When we walked into the expansive room, we were immediately hit with the pungent smell of formaldehyde. It's a smell that can turn your stomach. The combination of fluorescent light and that aroma made me immediately feel unwell on the first day. There were two rows of large silver tanks. Each one contained a human body. I couldn't help but look at each person and wonder what his or her story was.

We were given a woman as our cadaver. When we met

her, we all looked at her face. Our group decided to give her a name. We never wanted to be removed from the fact that she was a human being who was likely a wife, mother, grandmother, friend, colleague. We never wanted to look at this as a project; we wanted to see this as an amazing sacrifice from which we could learn and to become better physicians. Our group threw around ideas and eventually settled on 'Helen'.

I was in a group with young men who were amazing, intelligent, and kind. We all worked together to do the dissection and we would go over the anatomy time after time in an effort to make sure we all could get honors in this class. Every week we had new dissections to perform. Once the dissections were done, we would go from table to table to look at everyone else's dissections. It's a little-known fact that anatomy is fairly universal. However, every person has a slightly different appearance of the fine details. Each nuance is important. A surgeon especially should be exposed to as many as possible before operating on living people.

We were lucky to have the privilege of working as a team to educate each other. Also, having the honor of working with cadavers really changed some of my passions in medicine. I had never seen myself as a surgeon prior to the anatomy lab. It helped me gain confidence to do some of these detailed dissections alone. I will forever be grateful to my first patient, Helen. I began to realize that in death, there is also the link to life. In death, our stories aren't always over, and we can leave legacies that help people way into the future.

Am I a person or a lamp shade?

This was it, the show, the dance: the start of my clinical rotations as a medical student. I had never been more afraid of anything in my life. You hear horror stories about how medical students are treated. You worry about being able to go to the bathroom. You may not be able to eat before the day is done, which, let's be honest, breeds a very unhealthy relationship with food. Especially for those emotional eaters.

I knew there was no way I wanted to be an OBGYN. I thought, 'Holy smokes, their quality of life is horrific.' OB's are always on call, they're up at night, they seemed stressed. Knowing my personality, I would be chronically worried about outcomes and my high-risk patients. I just couldn't see myself part of that world.

So, what did I do? I fell in love with the one specialty I promised myself I would never pursue. I did my OBGYN rotation, second, after neurology. Everyone in the medical world says you should only do specialties early on that you know you don't want to have a career in. The reason? If you don't get honors it won't affect you when you are interviewing for residency programs.

The first time I ever set foot on labor and delivery, there was this adrenaline and nervous energy that was palpable. Within moments of arrival, a patient who was having her baby was wheeled past me and into a labor room. She spoke only Spanish and was screaming in pain. As a board certified OBGYN, I now know that scream, which is primal and visceral, it is the 'I am going to have a baby in the next two minutes' scream. I quickly walked bedside and put on gloves. The nurse called out as I walked in that she was going to deliver. As the baby was crowning, without anyone else in the room, I had a moment of terror, followed by excitement, joy, and happiness for this family. The attending and intern walked in as the head was delivering. Both started yelling at me as they got their gloves on. Before they were at my side the baby was out and laying comfortably on the mother. In that moment, I knew this was it; this was my specialty. In all the chaos, screaming, fear and anger, I was calm, steady and measured.

Everyone rotates through the specialties, regardless of their preference. I spent the remainder of my rotations trying to like everything else. I tried desperately to talk myself into pediatrics, general surgery, vascular surgery was amazing; let's be honest, any other specialty where you didn't have to wake up at 2:00 am on a regular basis and drive through unplowed snow-covered roads. The residency culture there also scared me. There was a chief resident who clearly hated her life and couldn't wait to take out her anger on every single resident and medical student below her. Now as a people pleaser obsessed with perfection, this was not an optimal match in personality.

Every morning I woke up by 4 a.m. and drove to the hospital. At that time, it's always dark in Wisconsin. Sometimes your eyes grow weary of the drive. However, when you are constantly in fluorescent lights and under scrutiny from every student, resident and attending in the hierarchy, the dark is a welcome respite. I would get there early, stay late, and try not to draw attention to myself. The other students advised me to listen, never talk first. I was so afraid someone would realize I wasn't qualified enough to be there. On some basic level, I think most doctors or doctors-in-training, medical students, and residents, will have imposter syndrome, this feeling that we are not meant to be there or that we don't deserve our place. We doubt that we are good enough to be trusted to care for patients. Coming from my background, this is something I struggled with a lot in early training. However, I felt that if I worked hard, then that hard work would be noticed and I wouldn't have to worry.

The problem in medicine is also that women don't always support other women. If a woman has had to fight her way to gain any sort of respect, there are some people who will openly and intentionally allow others to fail. This creates a malignancy like none other because you have men in a sick culture hoping people fail. Also, you have the very people you'd think to trust actively trying to minimize other women and their accomplishments, all so they can look better in the eyes of their male colleagues.

When I was going through training, the ACGME (Accreditation Council for Graduate Medical Education) was starting to say we should have work hour restrictions. However, while a good concept, you weren't ever going to be the person to bring this up. If you brought up how many hours you worked, you would be viewed as weak, lazy, and not a team player. We were also supposed to get four days off for the month in medical school. This means four days total for the month, including holidays, weekend days, Mondays, whatever days they wanted to give you. When you got those days off, you said thank you, and then you felt guilty taking them because inevitably someone would make passive-aggressive or aggressive-aggressive comments about medical students and their laziness. All this felt like more bait for women or men who were trying to make themselves look better or prove something to someone else.

When the time came to disclose which specialty I was going to pursue, I did some deep soul-searching. I set up a spreadsheet and entered data about what I loved about every specialty. I weighted them based on importance, and despite my best efforts to bias the data against OBGYN, that is what I ended up picking. I remember sitting with my vascular surgery attending, whom I loved, and was a force himself, and talking about my selection. He joked with me that he would still write me a letter of recommendation despite my poor decision to not go into surgery.

Picking a specialty is a leap of faith. I literally had to take out the malignant personalities from the OBGYN residency program to pursue this specialty. I loved everyone I worked with in surgery: the surgery residents, fellows, attendings; they were all able to be won over. I worked hard, I was smart, I was the first one to prep the lists, take off the bandages, pre-round, retract like a champion. They appreciated hard work. In OBGYN it felt like there was no winning, the culture was punitive, and if you stood out, the residents made you feel like you didn't belong.

I met with the OBGYN department chair and residency program director after I made my decision. In retrospect, it's hard to believe I used to be intimidated by anyone, but, of course, the chair was a gruff, very direct man who was known for 'pimping.' Yes, this sounds horrible if you're an outsider, but it means stopping in the middle of whatever task you are doing to ask questions repeatedly to the students or residents in an effort to 'educate.' Mostly, this approach just instils fear. In many cases, even if you know an answer, the manner in which the question is asked and the aggressive nature of the attending can render you frozen and unable to respond coherently. When I met with the residency director, he said he always liked me. He told me I was 'surprisingly smart.' His one complaint about me was that I was kind of like a 'lamp shade.' I looked at him with a healthy dose of intrigue stretched across my face.

'I was like a lamp shade?'

'Yeah, like in college, when you're at a party, you're like a lamp shade.'

'I'm not following. I guess I didn't go to a lot of parties.'

'You're quiet, you blend in, you're there, but not there. Most people might not notice the lamp. You need to speak up more. I hear you teaching other students how to read the strips (referring to fetal monitoring tracings), you should speak up more so we know what you're thinking.'

This entire conversation was so perplexing to me as a medical student. I'm supposed to be quiet, but loud, knowledgeable, but not so knowledgeable that the residents are made to look bad or less-than. I'm supposed to work hard, but not so hard that, again, the residents aren't angry I am there before them or show them up. I need to talk and tell people what I know, but I am, at my core, actually a shy person when it comes to bragging or showing people what I can do. I felt like working hard and doing my job, taking good care of patients should speak for itself. However, I found myself in a world where there were so many rules of conduct that I had no idea where to start to navigate the obstacles. Hmm, 'Lamp shade.' I just found that comment hilarious. Clearly these people didn't know me. But how would they know me? Did I want them to know me? I had grown up with a healthy distrust of anyone who had power over me. How would I navigate the sea of letting people close but not too close? Even now, when I am teaching, writing, or doing a speech, I look back and think, 'Who was that lamp shade girl?'

I went to Medical College of Wisconsin, in my biased opinion, the best medical school that exists in the world. It was tough, exhausting, emotionally depleting, and also provided the best education for me and my peers. You know I genuinely believe that if you can say all that about a school and still look back fondly at your formative years. As someone who has paid her way, medical school costs are daunting. During orientation, the spouses were invited to a financial discussion while we were doing something else. When we both emerged from our respective programs, my husband was thrilled to announce that, if I die, he won't have to pay back my loans. I looked at him with significant skepticism after his excited comment. Then I stopped and thought, 'Thank goodness, because if I die, I don't want my family crushed by $250,000 of debt.'

I didn't interview at many medical schools. I wanted to find a quality education first and foremost. However, I couldn't see myself moving from the Midwest. Unlike many of my peers, I didn't come from a wealthy background and certainly didn't have physicians in my family. I truly was going into medicine for the singular purpose of helping people. I wanted to live my life making a difference in other people's lives. I fully realized that decision may be somewhat to fill a need that I have always had, to be loved and valued, but still I felt like my life would be worthwhile if this is what I spent it doing. I worked feverishly to get myself into medical school. Despite the multitudes of people telling me not to do this, like an idiot, I still did it.

During my Honors banquet senior year at St. Mary's University of Minnesota, one of the professors I really looked up to, walked over to me after it was announced where we were going next year in terms of further education or work. He smiled sheepishly at me. I had known him for years, so that didn't make any sense. I started walking away and he called my name.

'Are you sure? Medical school?'

'Yup, it's what I've always wanted to do.'

'Really?'

'Yes, since I was four years old. I have wanted to do nothing else.'

'You know, it's going to be a long and hard road. Hope it's worth it for you.'

What was that supposed to mean? It felt so ominous. It felt like he was telling me I couldn't do it. I had so many people question whether I should be pursuing medicine. Not because they didn't think I could do it, but because they knew I wanted to have kids, or because I was a woman, or they were worried I couldn't deal with the malignant culture that came with medicine. They were worried that I wasn't tough enough to endure what I needed to get through to make it to the top of the mountain. If anyone knows anything about me, it's that if you tell me I can't do something, or act like I can't, I am going to be the first one to do it. I am going to be leading the medical school parade. If anything, all the cryptic messages furthered my resolve to continue on this path.

What's My Name?

I have never been called a bigger variety of names than when I started my medical career. I have to admit some of them have been my fault. Growing up I loved that my mother had a different last name than us kids. I felt like there was some anonymity when she would do things I didn't agree with. I never wanted to be judged for other's perceptions of my family. I wanted to be, singularly, critiqued by my own decisions and how I chose to treat people around me.

When I was a senior in college, I got engaged. I had just turned twenty-one the week before the proposal. I actually had my first official martini immediately following the blessed event. I have always been self-conscious, and it's true there were various times in my life where I had been in the limelight. I had a brief stint helping out with political campaigns. I introduced some pretty famous leaders when I was part of those campaigns. Despite that, I never liked the attention being on me or being around people who made judgments about my life with limited real data. So, on that day in October, we were at one my favorite jazz restaurants in the Twin Cities. I played alto saxophone and always loved jazz. My partner was acting so odd and he started making me anxious. At one point he spilled butter from the rolls onto my skirt. I immediately became fixated with the fact that I had this amazing suit skirt for my research presentations, and now there is this greasy butter stain for the world to see. He ended up getting frustrated with me and assured me we would get the marks out.

Between songs, he got up from his chair across from mine and proposed. All eyes were focused on us. Some people we didn't know were taking pictures. I, of course, said yes. I put the ring on and felt like the eyes were continually watching me as we sat there. I watched how the light reflected off my ring. In some way it felt like I had just been purchased, as odd as that sounds. I felt a little sick to my stomach. Where was I in this?

We called my dad shortly after to tell him about the engagement. He asked what my name would be? I said I wasn't sure.

'I guess I always thought you would be Dr. Lease.'

Well, that did it. Every time I thought about having one name, I heard the guilt from him and the husband. Unfortunately, I ended up with a long, but not really hyphenated name that confuses computer systems everywhere.

We planned our wedding for after my first year of medical school. This was to be the last summer with any time off during my education process. We settled on July 1st for the wedding date. Now, this date strikes fear in the hearts of every medical trainee. July 1st is the turnover date in medical school and residency. Logistically it made sense, but for almost a decade, our anniversary was one of the more traumatic days of the year.

My first day of residency, of course, was July 1st. We had finished our morning orientation and one of the chief residents were taking us on a brief tour of the units. She made sure we all had our badges to get in and out of locked stations. The stairwells also had codes for extra security. We all followed her around, wide-eyed, taking it in, scared that we were about to pretend to be physicians. We didn't know where to go or how to act. Most of us had never introduced ourselves as Dr. XYZ at that time. Your co-residents become your battle buddies. No one else understands all the dysfunction of your residency program or how you developed like your comrades.

The chief resident released most of the interns except myself and one other woman. She told us to go down and get changed into scrubs and come meet back at the resident lounge where she would be charting. Yes, this sounds like it should be the easiest request on planet earth. However, moments before, I had received a disgustingly large arrangement of flowers for my wedding anniversary, and I had nowhere to put them down. So, in my infinite wisdom, I decided to carry this display down the stairwell to the locker room.

I frantically dug through the scrub bins to come up empty handed, they only had small and extra small scrubs in the women's locker room. I could feel myself getting warm. Here I was, a physician, technically, I need to hustle to get back up to work, and I don't even have scrubs that will fit my 6'1", plus size self, and not only that, I am carrying this arrangement that is screaming of mediocrity. One of the guys in surgery was leaving his locker room, and with all my courage I had to yell at this very attractive young attending that I needed his help. He ran back into the men's locker room and pulled me medium scrub bottoms. I probably could have burst into tears in that moment. I wanted to scream down the hall, 'Do

I look like a size medium!' Well, I crammed all 6'1" into these pants, that were essentially high-water britches, and half my butt sticking out the top. Thank goodness for white coats to cover my tail end. I made my way back to the stairwell.

I ran up the stairs to the third floor and typed in, what I thought was my code. I am at this time, sweating, stressed, carrying a giant flower arrangement, and officially stuck in the stairwell with no idea how to contact anyone. So, I ran down to the first floor, again, code didn't work, ran up to the third floor, again code didn't work. At that moment, triage paged me overhead to come to triage. 'Dr. Stretcher to labor and delivery triage, Dr. Stretcher.' Just when I thought life couldn't get worse a second-year resident, who had a giant chip on her shoulder, and hated us interns, opened the door to see my anxious, sweaty self standing in the hallway. I pulled myself together, and I and my too-tight pants waddled to triage to see my first patient as an official physician.

In residency, you answer to whatever people call you. Stretcher, Stecher, Sticker, Lease Stecher, Kellie, Kell, Kells (my personal favorite), you there, girl, nurse, tech, dumbass, idiot, flirt, you get the point. You answer when you're called. Whatever you are called, it doesn't matter; you go, you work, you fix it, so you can move on.

As I progressed in my career, I realized most of those names don't go away. In fact, as a woman in medicine, I have been called far worse, especially when voicing an opinion that may not be similar to people in power.

Names matter, and what you call people matters. Addressing people appropriately and giving them respect sets the tone for good collegial relationships. It also helps to maintain patient safety. If you look at the evolution of medicine, men are usually immediately given respect. Upon entering a room, they are assumed to be the physician even when they aren't. In fact, the studies show male administrators and leaders who aren't physicians are treated with more respect than female physicians. I have been in meetings, spoken at conferences, been in operating rooms, and male physicians are addressed as Dr. X, while female physicians are addressed by their first names. Now, I firmly believe in breaking down barriers to communication. I think errors in healthcare can be decreased when you don't have such a strong hierarchy, but how is it that in the 21st century men are still treated with more respect than women?

Research supports that when women stop using their credentials, they are less likely to have leadership positions, less likely to be taken seriously, not given promotions, paid less, and become less involved. All these things contribute to physician burn out. Recent policy changes that were created by men, suggested we go by first names. Not shockingly, the men are still called doctor while the women are treated very casually. Even in basic day to day ads for corporations, women are called by their first name or first and last, and men are addressed as Dr. X. Names matter, respect matters, treating people as people matters. When it comes to a name, everyone needs to have the same standards across all of healthcare.

Women in healthcare also need to be keenly aware of who owns them. They are, in fact, their own brand. No one should have rights to who you are, what you think, or what your name is. I had to spend time gaining rights to my own name on google. It was through those lessons I realized I won't let anyone control any facet of who I am professionally or personally. Oprah used to tell people to not let anyone write blank checks under her name. In today's digital culture and competition, don't let anyone control anything with your name. You need to know what's going out into the world and what you are associated with. If different projects don't serve to further your energy, beliefs, and motivations, then they need to be evicted from your life .

Time of Death…

Doctors go through incredible challenges which changes them, in both positive and negative ways. We spend eighty plus hours a week with some of our co-workers during training. Every waking moment is dedicated to the practice of medicine. When we graduate medical school, we are technically doctors, and we get the two initials behind our name MD. However, it is with every moment we practice we earn those letters, like a merit badge.

In residency, we are all expected to rotate through the ICU. Some of us rotate in the surgical or medical ICUs, while others have the misfortune of rotating through both, depending on what your specialty demands.

In the intensive care units, you see things that, as an OBGYN, you really hope not to encounter frequently. In the OBGYN world, most of the time, the story has a happy ending. However, when things go bad, they can go bad fast. It is for that reason that we are expected to get our ICU training.

When I was on rotation, I did central lines, art lines, and intubations. I basically did whatever I was told to do; that's what you do in medicine. When someone says run, you run. Did I want to do any of those things? No, not in the slightest. However, I realized a long time ago that, to make forward progress in life and to grow as a physician, you need to get comfortable with being uncomfortable.

There are certain rites of passage from which no one in training is immune. We all know these things are coming; we just don't know when, where or how. On a random Tuesday night intern year, while on call, one of the ICU nurses paged me..

'Dr. Stretcher?'

'Yes.' You noticed that I just respond to whatever they called me. Strecher, Stryker, Streaker, I was in the ICU for four to six weeks. They weren't going to bother to learn my name. I already tried down that road.

'The patient I am taking care of has died.'

In this situation, it was a patient who said 'Do Not Resuscitate (DNR)'; we were making him comfortable. The family was aware and given time to say goodbye. It was a situation that seemed slightly more palatable than when we lose someone instantly and by surprise. I put my big girl pants on and mustered the strength to go into the room where the family was sitting, holding their loved ones' hands. The room was dark and eerily silent. Most of the ICU rooms were full of noise and chaos because of the machines dinging and IV poles beeping. To walk into a room full of people that has no movement and no sound is heartbreaking.

The nurse handed me the stethoscope. You could tell she was annoyed I needed to come. The ICU nurses have been doing this forever, and now here was an OBGYN intern coming in to make the proclamation. I listened to his chest and watched for the rise and fall out of instinct. I could feel his body was already rigid from everything he had gone through. My eyes met his widow's. It's as if, without saying a thing, my eyes betrayed me, and told her the truth before my mouth could. She grabbed the handkerchief from the nightstand and patted tears away. I looked back at the clock.

'Time of death....'

Another Day Another Dollar

Physicians go through a constant evolution of personal and professional catastrophes. As it turns out, we have a higher rate of suicide, depression, and anxiety. Female physicians are at risk of burn out at alarming rates . I believe the higher rate of burn out among female physicians is because we are, to a large extent, empaths. We constantly are working to help others. It is exhausting. Unlike men, we don't get recognized as much for awards or leadership positions. We are in situations where we are punished for the same things men would be rewarded for.

I have been trusted with the stories of many who have walked the road toward becoming a physician. These women are strong, persistent, determined and, in many cases, fearless, except for the concern about losing their hard-earned jobs. These women are more scrutinized than their male counterparts. If they take a more direct tone of voice, they are written up, despite men in some institutions being allowed to yell, scream, and throw adult tantrums at anything that moves.

My female colleagues across the country tell the same stories. It's not uncommon for someone to need to move forward with an urgent surgery, and at that time force a male surgeon to wait for an elective case. Often, these women physicians are ostracized because they have inconvenienced a man. The narrative is regularly, 'Who is this young woman doctor? She had the audacity to make a middle aged, white surgeon wait to do his elective case?' These moments happen every day. These moments take away the joy women experience when they take care of their patients.

Between increasing patient loads, providing amazing care, insurance shortcomings for patients, call burdens, administrative duties, licensing requirements, continued education, involvement as faculty, and leaders in the community, women shouldn't have the added burden of proving themselves to everyone every day of their lives. They should be treated with the same respect that their male counterparts are naturally shown. A man shouldn't be believed to be honest, ethical or just, simply because he happens to be a man. However, the same should hold true of women. No one has ever suggested that a woman be given better opportunities or treatment. We all know that wouldn't happen. No, we just want to be seen, heard, treated with dignity, and considered in the narrative.

The studies have long showed that women physicians are actually amazing at their jobs. We are usually extremely self-critical, communicate more easily, and don't rely on extreme hierarchical issues. For these reasons, patient care is often done in a safer fashion. Staff feel more comfortable talking to us about their concerns and patient needs.

As you can imagine, the armor we wear every day needs to be tough and have resiliency so we can be our best selves for our patients. However, when we go into battle to do what is right for our community, we need more allies and less adversaries. Otherwise, we are wasting bullets on people who don't deserve our time.

It's just PCOS and a little infertility...

Most people start making life plans when they're fairly young. I knew I wanted to be a mom and a doctor when I was four-years-old. Funnily enough, my daughter has made the same comments. It's obvious I need to be putting more money into my kids' education funds.

When I got to my teenage years, my pediatrician also thought my height might be problematic in regard to my fertility. He referred me to an endocrinologist in the 'big city,' Madison, WI. I was in my early teen years, so I didn't have a license. My father and I made the journey to Madison together. When we arrived, we parked, walked in, checked in and I was so embarrassed to be there with my dad, I probably said three words to him the entire time.

When they called my name, they somehow made 'Kellie' sound like they had never said the name before, 'Keeley.' I looked at my dad, 'You think that's me?'

The receptionist pointed at me and we walked into the back as my dad sat reading magazines in the waiting room. I remember the smell as we walked through the halls. It seemed like a mixture of stale, burned coffee, and Lysol. It was almost enough to knock you off your feet. Everything also seemed brighter and harsher. I went to school at a very sterile place, and somehow, this seemed like a more aggressive environment. For the first time in a long time, I felt truly anxious.

I really didn't know why the pediatrician referred me to the endocrinologist. The only experience I had had with them was my grandmother who checked her blood sugars multiple times a day for diabetes. The medical assistant checked my blood pressure, took down my weight, and handed me a gown that opened to the front. I had never taken my pants off for an appointment, so I looked perplexed by the gown. She smiled when she saw my face.

'You only need to take off your top and bra.'

I instantly got a migraine. What is the point of taking off my top? I whipped my top off as fast as possible and threw on the gown. I wasn't going to be the girl half naked when the doctor walked in. Of course, I had to tuck my bra into my shirt, as if I was fooling anyone that the bra existed.

I sat on the examination table staring at the wall on which there was a picture of a hot air balloon. I couldn't help but wish I was in the basket of the balloon, floating away from whatever conversation I was about to have.

When the doctor walked in, his eyes never left the paper chart. He was flipping through the labs that had been sent over from my doctor. He mumbled something inaudibly under his breath and walked to my side. He placed the cold stethoscope on my bare skin, which during winter in Wisconsin, also seemed like a bridge too far.

'Deep breath, again, again, let it out.'

He pulled up the gown to look at my chest. Now, as a physician, I realize why he did that. He was looking at breast development, hair patterns, fat deposition, etc. As a 13-year-old child, given no explanation, it felt very intrusive.

'So, as it turns out you have something called PCOS. You have hyperandrogenism. You are likely to have trouble getting pregnant. There are medications we can put you on to help. We could put you on medication now, depending on a couple follow up results. So, we will get more labs today and you can see an endocrinologist closer to home next time.'

Well, with that I was left in the harsh reality that I might be infertile or I might not. Did I have some elevated hormone? I got my top back on and went to the lab. When I got in the car. I was quiet and staring out the window. Dad asked how it went. 'I don't know, I may have problems having kids in the future.'

After that appointment I spent many years wondering if I would be able to have kids. I have had patients with the same diagnosis made to think they could never get pregnant, and have accidental pregnancies because they have chosen to not be on birth control. Communication is key to everything in life, especially where kids are concerned.

The puppy, a trailer park, and October nights

Medical school and Residency are breeding grounds for feelings of depression and inadequacy. When I started residency, all my co-residents and I trauma-bonded from fear of what was to come. It's a pretty dramatic lifestyle and cultural change to go from school to actually being a physician, even if it is just training.

I was not feeling my usual self. I was frustrated I didn't get things as easily. It was like, for the first time in a long while, I was worked to exhaustion. Because of my clear malaise and the fact that I had found mice in our apartment, I was trying to force my husband to get out of the nine months remaining on our lease; he decided the lesser of the evils would be to allow me to get a dog.

My persistence at requesting a fury baby had finally paid off. Lucky for him, I had been secretly doing research about what breeds I wanted, what made sense with our space, budget and long-term living situation. I decided, due to size restrictions, I obviously couldn't get the giant Bernese Mountain Dog that I dreamed about. However, I found a breed that I thought would be perfect, non-shedding, small, really affectionate: a Cavachon, Cavalier and Bichon Frise mix. I also tracked down a place that sold them near us in Michigan.

My husband called the breeder and, to my excitement, we found out they had a litter that was ready to go home.

One October evening we loaded up the car and made the trek about an hour away from Grand Rapids. I had convinced him we wouldn't be getting the dog that night and would just look and see if he or she seemed like the right fit.

The sun had set by the time we got close to the home. It gave off an eerie haunted house type of feeling as we drove along the path. I called one of my girlfriends and told her the address in case we disappeared, since we had gotten this information off an online advert. I could see the headline now: resident and husband, giant idiots, went into the middle of nowhere to get a dog that didn't exist, didn't come home.

When we got to the address, there was a little trailer home. We knocked and went inside. They had many dogs crammed into a tiny area. All the new puppies were behind a baby gate in the living room. The room had torn up, matted green carpet. It smelled like the entire floor was painted in urine. As we stood there, an adult dog relieved himself in the middle of the floor.

'That's the puppy's daddy.' The lady yelled down the hall.

I looked at Joe and he knew exactly what I was thinking.

'NO! Just one!'

'But... how on earth can I leave the other four!?'

'No, just one!'

I started getting anxious thinking about getting one. Why is one better than the other. Why would one be able to escape tonight and not the other ones. I immediately started feeling guilty because I couldn't take them all with me.

They opened the gate and let the five puppies stumble around. They were all so sweet and fluffy and loving. I initially picked up a little girl who was feisty, fearless, and full of energy. Joe immediately didn't like that one, which is hilarious now since that is my daughter's and my personality. Clearly, he was happy we weren't stuck with a puppy version of us as well.

There was a shy little boy who came over to me and asked to be picked up. I put him on my lap and he nuzzled into me. That was it, and I was in love. Patrick Atticus Stecher, got sprung and became our furry baby.

Having a dog in residency was the best thing that I possibly could have done. I rushed home to see him. He made me exercise outside. He slept with me when I was on night float so I didn't feel alone 24/7. I think it's really important for physicians-in-training to find whatever thing, whether its exercise or a pet, to help them feel more human during training.

Mom

When I was a chief resident, I figured we should start trying for me to get pregnant. As an OBGYN resident, I was fairly convinced I would need some sort of infertility therapy and, at the very least, necessitate medication management. I kept hearing the words of the endocrinologist I had seen. PCOS, which is polycystic ovarian syndrome, does make it harder to conceive. In retrospect, I'm surprised that, at my age and symptoms, that's the diagnosis they came up with.

Residency isn't for the faint of heart; it's monumentally difficult, and that's for a clear reason. You need to be prepared to handle anything at any time, even when you are at near-death exhaustion levels. I started feeling more run-down, just fatigued in general. I had constant muscle aches and more headaches which I attributed to being a chief on a service.

Since I am a terrible patient, as most physicians and nurses are, I had already determined I should meet with a reproductive endocrinologist. I saw a physician with whom I worked and respected. He was a tall, lanky, somewhat nerdy man, who's Diet Coke obsession rivalled mine. My husband and I went in for the consult. Our doctor asked the typical questions and talked about testing. We went over my menstrual cycles. I was talking about how they were more regular with weight-loss and working out, and then he asked when my last menstrual period was.

In that moment, I felt like the worst OBGYN in the world. I couldn't tell him my LMP. I think six or so weeks ago. My husband let out the loudest sigh of annoyance.

'Huh, what if you're pregnant now. Maybe we should take a pregnancy test.' My husband wasn't playing.

I couldn't help but acknowledge that as a somewhat realistic possibility. I mean, we had been trying; nothing was working. I had made the appointment and quit tracking and trying. The pregnancy test was, in fact, positive that day. A few hours later my attending called and asked me to come in for an ultrasound the next day. It was so sweet; he came in on a Saturday morning so we could figure out what my dating was.

When the picture came on the screen, I could see my little peanut. I always thought they looked like gummy bears at that stage of the game. There was my little guy, all seven weeks of him, with a perfect little heartbeat and no areas of bleeding; all was healthy. The second time we tried for pregnancy we used some medical assistance with medication and ovidrel, which forces you to ovulate, and then we had my daughter. We were blessed with my little people, and very lucky they have completed our family.

No use crying over spilled milk...

Having a newborn can be very challenging for new families. I try to mentally prepare my patients especially for the first two weeks. At the time of writing the world is in the grip of a declared Pandemic. We know that the stress of this will add a dramatic increase of cases of postpartum depression and anxiety as well. Women struggling with being new moms, breastfeeding, balancing work and life, are now often facing the challenges in a more isolated fashion. When I was postpartum, all I wanted was my sister to come over and sit with me for support. Whatever the reason, being cut off from your normal social support poses more challenges.

After I had my son, Joseph, we were fairly isolated because we lived in Michigan, and away from our family. I had pre-eclampsia with him and was induced at 35+6 weeks gestation. Your due date is 40 weeks. My poor little man was 5 lbs. 11 oz when we left the hospital, and he had reflux, jaundice, and was a cranky colicky guy.

After he was born, I felt like a failure that I couldn't keep him in longer. I did everything I could do to keep my blood pressures down, I was taking labetalol every four hours, even waking up at night, and nearing maximum doses. To put that in perspective, usual dosing of Labetalol is twice a day. However, despite my efforts, pregnancy presents a challenge to the body that is often a losing battle. This is the case with most pregnancy associated complications. If you have gestational diabetes and need insulin, often your insulin requirements will further increase through the pregnancy.

I was going to one of my twice-weekly prenatal appointments and standing in line to check in when I started having visual changes and a severe headache. I looked at Joe and told him I was definitely going to the hospital and being delivered that day. Pre-eclampsia with severe features has an unmistakable feeling, and it felt peculiar that I was experiencing the symptoms that I had discussed with thousands of patients.

I was admitted into the hospital and was assessed in the triage area. Butterworth Hospital felt like a second home to me, with my friends and attendings all in one place. I was started on magnesium sulfate for seizure prophylaxis. I felt like a drunk sailor, riding on a ship engulfed in tidal waves. I was hot, sweaty, nauseas, dizzy, and couldn't focus my attention on anything. The Maternal Fetal Medicine physician, whom I loved, came to check on me and to offer a primary cesarean section since I was starting out with a closed cervix. Sadly, I declined the offer because I thought I had a great chance at getting a tiny pre-term baby out of my vagina. After all, I told myself the lie many women tell themselves, I had wide hips which should mean good for birthing.

After a day of medication and induction, my blood pressures became more severe. I had a moment where I lost consciousness and my husband consented for a cesarean section. The next thing I recall is being wheeled into the operating room and my amazing friends and OBGYNs were there to deliver my son. As soon as I heard him cry, I honestly thought to myself, 'He's good; it's totally ok if I am not now.' I recovered from surgery and pre-eclampsia amazingly well. I also decided to give breastfeeding my best shot.

Breastfeeding is something I lovingly refer to as the worst part of having a newborn. Regardless of who you are or what your background is, you have likely been told of the benefits of breastfeeding. Now, as a physician, I know that the medical literature supports breastfeeding, and I was all-in on this endeavor. Those who know me know I can be rather compulsive once I put my mind to something, and I don't stop until I get the project done.

Breastfeeding was something I approached with that same mentality. Of course, my tiny, colicky, jaundiced newborn didn't want to latch or cooperate. I remember trying to fit my entire areola in his mouth, to get a good latch, and thinking this looks like James and the Giant Peach. I kept putting my hand by his nose because I was convinced I was suffocating him. It was actually hard the first few weeks because when we fed him supplemental breastmilk, or my breastmilk from a bottle, he was so thin you could feel it going down his esophagus into his stomach.

Every morning, we would wake up and give ourselves a mental pat on the back that we survived another day as parents. We tried the supplemental feeder, pumping more, expressing milk, nipple shields; we went so far as to try this rather uncomfortable device that sucked my nipples out further so he might get more to latch onto. The weeks went fast, and when I returned to work, I was on my GYN Oncology rotation. Sadly, this may have been the worst rotation to come back from postpartum on, but you can't choose when life happens. I remember standing during a ten-hour surgery, and my breasts got rigid hard. I could feel the milk leaking down my chest and stomach. I was so intent on the surgery I didn't even know that I had leaked through my scrub top and gown until the tech told me. Once I got home, I was in so much pain I pumped as quickly as I could at top speed. From that moment on the milk supply tanked.

However, with my daughter it was an entirely different story. In my mind I had a direct plan of attack for breastfeeding. I was going to pump right away, a supplemental feeder was purchased, she was going to be delivered at term. I was convinced I could make this work. With her I had such an oversupply she couldn't keep up, and it was like I was water boarding her.

What do you do with a crazy oversupply? Well, you pump and save the milk so you can donate the breastmilk to babies who need it. I filled our freezer, the basement freezer, and a full chest freezer in the garage, and realized I needed to figure out the breastmilk donation process. I came across a website, 'Human Milk For Human Babies', a kind of a Craig's list for breastmilk. I scrolled through the stories and names and found this amazing family who had had twins. Their beautiful mom was recently diagnosed with cancer and couldn't produce enough breastmilk for them. Well, we gave it a shot and set up the milk exchange. I brought all my std testing and prenatal labs, as many viruses can cross into breastmilk and I wanted them to have full disclosure. I was able to give them milk until they were a year old. I was honored to get to go to the birthday party with my daughter and son. I also gave milk to a little guy who was adopted and occasionally supplemented milk for a pre-term baby.

I tell my patients no two pregnancies are the same, and that is true for the postpartum period as well. Everyone who has had children knows they need all the kindness and support they can get. We also need to look out for each other and the crazy high expectations that we put on ourselves and other people to be this perfect mom. No one is perfect. You need to find whatever way you want to parent. You just need to be happy with what you're doing, and how you're taking care of your little peanut.

The Girl Who Lived

I was young, well, younger than I am now, and I was newly in private practice, when I felt like I made it to the mountain top. I was slowly getting into the new rhythm of life that comes with being a full time OBGYN and mother. Up until that point, the only dream I had was becoming a doctor, then an OBGYN, then getting all my board certifications. When you pour your entire life and soul into a career, which many of us would say is more of a calling, the rest of your life disappears. You work hard to make it through the next challenge, pass by the next obstacle.

When I had started in practice, it was a small three-woman clinic that went to two different hospitals. When I had signed my contract, I had been promised I would only be going to one location, and as a new graduate, I only really wanted to have one to focus all my attention on. However, that didn't work out, and somehow, I think I managed the changes as well as could be expected. I was a busy clinician; I was working through any of the anxieties I had about starting my career.

I gave birth to my daughter early in my time at the private practice. I was able to take off eight weeks after my Cesarean section. To me, as someone who loved her patients and missed the work, that felt like a long time away. I fully realize for many twelve, sixteen, thirty weeks or even a lifetime wouldn't be enough time to be home with a newborn, but it felt doable.

88

Kellie Lease Stecher, MD

Twelve weeks would have been preferable, but I didn't have that luxury.

The way I take care of my patients allows me to become an interloper in their families. I follow my patients, I see them for appointments, review ultrasounds with them, and am there nine out of ten times for their deliveries. This has given me such satisfaction in my job. I tell all my infertility patients that the happiest I am is when I can help them achieve a pregnancy and deliver their baby.

There was one family who became near and dear to my heart and soul. They were stuck coming in frequently because of a twin pregnancy. They had other beautiful children. They were rooted and grounded in love for each other. My patient was, in fact, a twin herself. She was as close to her twin as any sister could be. They were actually both pregnant at the same time and delivered shortly after I came back from maternity leave. I knew I couldn't miss being a part of the delivery of her babies.

In the obstetric world, we deal with many emergencies. Of course, during the pregnancy, we are constantly thinking about how the baby is growing, anatomically how is the baby, what risk factors moms could have for the pregnancy or delivery. There isn't a second of the pregnancy that your OBGYN isn't thinking about how to make sure you and the baby/babies are safe. We try to reduce your risk of transfusion after delivery by making sure you take your iron and correct anemia. We check your blood pressure and look for any signs of increased swelling to the point of concern that could be signs of pre-eclampsia or hypertension issues that could affect you and the baby.

The mental check list of prenatal care is endless. Twins, however, add one more nuance to the care. That nuance is providing counseling and planning for delivery. During the course of a twin pregnancy, we plan for every scenario that could happen. We talk through all the surprises, baby positioning, the risks of potential need for emergency interventions, NICU, or even death.

On that particular day, I had a rather ominous feeling. I knew I wouldn't be doing the delivery alone because I don't do breech vaginal deliveries. I had my senior partner with me to make sure things went smoothly. Her son, twin A, third of her sons, was born with barely a hiccup of a push. He was beautiful and perfect and sweet. When I went to feel for her daughter she was still not positioned ideally. I stepped aside and let my partner work. Events took place that then had us doing an emergency Cesarean section. In my mind, every moment is as clear as the day it happened. I know where I was standing, which nurses were watching and waiting. I know my demeanor and tone during the process. I can feel the goosebumps on the back of my neck when my partner didn't get her delivered. She came out and was beautiful but quiet. The NICU team quickly did their job. and she was transferred to the University for more intensive care.

I drove home, crying the entire way, as I didn't have a good feeling about this situation. I walked into my daughter's nursery. I looked at my beautiful, perfect, sleeping angel, and rocked her for three hours. I cried over her body and snuggled her tight. In my irrational postpartum, grieving mind, I felt guilt. Why is my child in my arms and hers is in the NICU? Maybe I should give her Addie? What if she loses her first daughter? This was, in fact, the first big struggle of patient care I had ever had. The way we provide care made it even harder on me. Remember, I felt like I knew these people. I was part of their lives, even if it was just for a moment.

The next day, I went to see her in her hospital room. I walked in, sat next to her, and we hugged and cried together. We transferred her to the other hospital so she could be near the baby. Every day, I would talk to the NICU physicians. Some days, the news was better than others. There was a moment where I knew it couldn't be a good outcome, and I took the call from a patient room. I remember him talking to me calmly and slowly, trying to articulate everything for me. Each word I took directly into my heart. Each word caused me anguish. I sat down on the exam table and cried. I couldn't believe that, in this world, doing everything we could, trying our best, taking all the precautions, this would happen. I didn't know if I wanted to be an OBGYN anymore. I wanted to leave, hang up my stethoscope, and walk out the back door.

My senior partner acted annoyed that I considered taking a day off work and that I was affected by the situation. I went to visit my patient at the NICU, my friend and partner came with me and stayed in the hallway so I could see the family. She stood in the hall, like a guardian angel, making sure we were there for support.

The day of the funeral, I made it to their church. When I got out of the car, I immediately was tearful. The day was crisp, and slightly cloudy. I was invited, of course, or I wouldn't have come. However, in that moment, I didn't feel like I deserved to be there. I had bought her a necklace with her daughter's initial. I did this so she could have a little object to touch close to her heart that would remind her of her daughter. Hopefully, she could feel her with her always in everything she did and know what an amazing mother she was to her boys.

When the funeral was over, we all went outside and held purple balloons. The family gave the most beautiful speech. During the speech, her husband talked about me, and they thanked me, and in that moment, they saved me. We launched the balloons into the heavens to celebrate this sweet girl that we wouldn't get to hold again.

In her death, she saved me. I was surrounded by the most beautiful family. My work colleagues I loved like sisters sat beside me. I saw what true unconditional love was, a love that was omnipresent and had no bounds or ending. In that moment, I met a little more of myself, the part that could let go. The part that was going to release the sadness into heaven, and clear my head, and move on to take care of my family and my patients. In her death, I began to love more completely and at my core. I began to lean into the good, bad, ugly, whatever it was. I learned that you need to be there to show people love, kindness, and compassion.

There were times in my life where I had been scared to lean in. I had been scared to make myself vulnerable and open. I was scared to be honest with my feelings. I think all of that is fairly natural bearing in mind the environment I had come from.

My patient sent me purple roses after the funeral. I brought them home from work and showed my newborn daughter. I told her about her friend, her guardian angel. I gave her the roses, seemed fitting since her name is Addison Rose.

When she had her next baby, I was there by her side. And because my partner knew the story he was there by mine. Of course, everything went well. But sometimes it's nice to have a guardian angel on earth. And, just like that, my healing started.

A Wedding and a Psychic

In the last few years, I have realized that you shouldn't ask questions that you don't want answered. I have countless patients who will call at night or during the day for reassurance, which I totally get. However, if I am worried about you, I am going to send you into the clinic to be seen or the hospital to be evaluated. Sometimes those patients aren't happy with me that they need to be seen; however, in those cases I may be worried about a multitude of things that we often can't diagnose over the phone and, at the very least, can't treat adequately. As a physician, you would think I would have learned those very lessons myself. However, we don't like to take our own medicine.

A few years ago, we flew into Arizona for my brother and sister-in-law's destination wedding. It was beautiful, the scenery was lovely, it was great weather, and everything went off without any major issues. Of course, we had little hiccups, as any wedding might do. Addie, who was flower girl, fell over and skinned her face the day before the ceremony and one of the bridesmaids somehow turned herself green because of a combination of sunscreen and perfume.

Kristen, my sister, and I needed to essentially crush each other into our dresses to make them zip and look nice. I have to say, for the first time in my life, I was feeling fierce because I had lost that 150 pounds. I was feeling so grateful because if there was ever a time to be near a goal weight, it was when someone was going to pay for a professional photographer.

Before the ceremony, I had a genius idea. I decided we should all go to a psychic for individual readings. If anyone should have put the kibosh on this, it should have been my sister, who is very logical. However, the train had left the station, and we were on route to this psychic.

We pulled up to this rather non-descript building that had an industrial flare. It looked as though no one was there for these readings that were allegedly 'the best in Sedona.' We stood on the stoop waiting for signs of movement. I thought this could not possibly be a very good psychic because she should surely know we're standing here and anticipate our needs. I had never been to a psychic. I didn't have any previous interest. I didn't give any weight to energies or soulmates or soul connections.

I kept hearing the wind chimes on the door. It was actually quite lovely; it sounded like the same chimes my grandma and Grandpa Lease had had at their front door. The lady saw us and let us in. I guess she had been doing an in-home reading, whatever that meant. We all piled into the seating area, which had the typical psychic layout with a bonsai tree and water fountain. She took each of us into our readings individually.

When it was my turn, it felt very somber. Honestly, I felt like I was about to go talk to a priest or get into trouble. She sat across from me and had me hold out my hands.

'Hmmmm.'

The silence was not entertaining. She touched an area on my palm and began speaking.

'You see here. Here is another great love. Hmmm. But with love comes change. You aren't in your forever job.'

'No, I think I'm good.'

She looked at me and raised an eyebrow. 'No, you're not in your forever job. You will do something where you can use more of your talents.'

I'm fairly certain I rolled my eyes. What other talents did I have? I worked my entire life to be an OBGYN, so what did that comment mean?

'Do you mean not in medicine?'

'No, not necessarily, you will just be somewhere where you can use your other talents to help people. You can use what you do now and what you want in the future. But I see a tower, a fall, and a big change. I see a soul contract that can't be broken.'

'What's a soul contract?'

'You have another soulmate; you've lived other lifetimes knowing them. You are supposed to engage in this life together as well. There will be a big fall with this person.'

When I left, I really didn't feel that I had been entertained the way I expected. Instead, I felt very depressed and not sure what to make of it. I was fairly certain she was making things up for me. Everyone started sharing their readings which all seemed to make sense for them. Apparently, everyone was going to live happily ever after. But I was going to take some fall from a tower, with some soul contract and new job. Whatever... There is value in listening to what you want, and not living a life other people think you should. I'll maybe just stick to that plan.

A girl and her Mustang

L ife is made up of a thousand little endings and beginnings. We are, in fact, the only main character who remains constant throughout the architecture of our lives. When I was younger, I had friends who had parents with motorcycles and convertibles. I thought that driving one of those would be as close as I could come to flying on earth. Like many physicians, especially the ones who operate, there is an element of risk-taking and adrenaline-seeking that is part of how we are made up. We deal with life and death, as cliché as that is.

There are many of us that medicate the stress of our jobs with dating, alcohol, or even substance abuse. We are in school and training for the vast majority of our prime young years. Many of us sacrificed our late teens and early twenties to get into school. So, what do we do? We find different outlets to create distractions from daily life.

Of course, some people transition smoothly from one event to the next. Some physicians have amazing healthy boundaries where they are at work, totally checked into what they are doing, and once they leave, they can change gears immediately. I, on the other hand, was never someone who could turn off my mind. I can always find one more project to complete, one more patient to worry about, one more plan to make, one more event or conference to speak at or attend.

I was never one to be happy with second place or a close finish, I was in constant need to be better than... the next whatever it may be. I didn't realize that I had turned into my own malignant competitor. I had evolved into a person that couldn't enjoy little things in life. I didn't take time to go to games or watch a new TV series.

Then it happened. I met a friend who made me realize what I was missing. She totally understood me, in my head, the job, all of it. This friend was able to make me see color in life. She made me feel like there was a steady flow to the water, and, potentially, I could stop searching for more, often the unattainable. I became fine treading water and taking moments to enjoy life. To some that may seem ridiculous, but for someone who had never been anchored, this was a significant breach of the forcefield of my own making.

I was inspired to get the car I always wanted. I picked up my sister, who was forever my partner in crime, and forced her to go with me to the dealership. There is something about a solitary woman entering a car dealership that weirded me out. I walked in and wanted to test drive the Ford Mustang that I had seen online. The dealership was slow. I think there was one other customer mulling around the vehicles. One of the male workers came over and asked if my husband would be along.

'Nope, just us.'

'Will he need to sign?'

'Nope, I got it.'

'Are you able to get a loan?'

'Yes, I am.'

'Oh, what do you do?'

'I'm a doctor.'

With that lovely icebreaker all conversation stopped.

Another salesperson - a woman - came over. She helped us right away, and we bought my car that I had wanted for all my life. When I picked it up, I put the top down, and drove it off the lot myself.

There is something empowering to someone, (like me) who couldn't afford to go to camp, but then can buy the car you always wanted and drive it away, having paid with money you alone earned. When I pulled onto the highway, I knew that that was as good as it got. In that moment, I was fine, my kids were fine, my job was great, I felt like I had renewed faith in men and humankind. The problem with having it all is that things don't equal happiness. Before I drove home, I of course had to share this moment with my friend. After all, what is life without people to share special moments with? When we don't have people we love in our lives, it really does drain the color from every second of every day.

There was a summer not long ago where I was transitioning jobs. It was stressful and overwhelming. I was back to focusing on survival. The color was gone out of every moment. I would wake up, get dressed, go to work, function in a near mechanical way to put one foot in front of the other. I was probably five percent the person I wanted to be. I was going through significant personal changes and didn't know how to balance being a mom and physician during this time.

There were nights when I would walk through the door and go right to bed. I was so depleted from everything going on around me and in my life. I seemed unable to take one more thing from anyone. My sister came over one night as I laid in the dark, in my room, crying into a pillow. I was actively wishing I didn't exist. She held my hand and laid next to me for hours until I fell asleep. She then started making plans for how to help me get through this phase of life, to help me end this chapter so I could get to the new beginning she knew I needed. Each day became an unbearable burden. I felt alone and isolated and I grieved for the life that I had lost.

Slowly, though, as the days went on, I was able to smile and regain some joy in the little things. I remember it had been months that I hadn't put the top down on my convertible. As I was leaving clinic, I pressed the button to retract the roof, and as the air hit my face as I cruised along the highway, it was like I could taste the sun, I was beginning to find joy in life once more. I finally found some color left in the few pieces that remained of the person I was. I picked up the shards of shattered glass that was my life and watched the light from the sun make them into something else entirely.

Don't Let Someone Else Mold You

I n the quiet moments before I walk into the hospital, I try to still my thoughts. However, in these instants, when I am alone in my car, ready to start a day, I hear the words that have been said in an effort to cut me down. I hear the words used to dismiss me, to devalue me, to make me worthless in someone else's eyes. The problem is, I can still hear the voices of many people who tried to crush my sense of self-worth and my dreams. I have tried almost everything; working out, eating better, meditation. I have tried focusing all off-work time on my kids. I have seen a therapist to deal with trauma that continue to haunt me.

Why do women need to do this in the workplace? Why can some men get away with lying and trying to ruin someone else's career? Is it because there are no safeguards in medicine? Why are too few willing to say that this behavior is unacceptable? There is no governing body that put an end to abuse or harassment women face in the workplace each day.

If women challenge those who are engrained in the medical culture, women in medicine are looked at as disruptive. We are questioned about motives and are not taken seriously. Many people pay us lip service that they agree no one should have this power over us, but no one does anything actionable. In fact, nothing changes. When I have tried to be an active part of systemic transformation, I have been told: 'culture is hard to change.'

We watch countless women, such as physicians, that are highly intelligent, and great at their jobs, leave medicine or become depressed, anxious, or suffer PTSD caused as a direct result of inappropriate interactions with male colleagues, yet no one will start to change the culture. Despite proposal after proposal, much talk comes to little or nothing. Why? Because there is inertia. What happens, happens; boys will be boys, they didn't mean what they did, you're too sensitive, you are clearly overemotional. No one should be threatened in the workplace, not least physicians who have made significant sacrifices throughout their entire lives to earn the jobs they have and to fight to be heard and treated as equals.

I was in a surgeons' lounge, the only woman present. In only a ten-minute interval, multiple things happened that made me uncomfortable. One of the men shushed me and said, 'Kellie, quiet. Men are talking.'

This was when I was offering a different perspective on something I had every right to have an opinion. I also was told that I had intentionally put my 'ass in Dr. X's face.'

To survive, what do you do? You make a joke, 'If I wanted to put my ass in your face there wouldn't be any ambiguity about it.'

I would love to say this was a gross departure from reality; however, these were non-malignant interactions. In these moments at least the men were laughing.

As women, what do we want? We want to be taken seriously as physicians and colleagues. We want a seat at the table. We want to work hard. We want to take care of our patients. We want to be successful in our fields. How do we do that? Often, it is through playing someone else's game. A game that you wouldn't even recognize yourself.

It's hard for people outside of medicine to truly grasp how far behind the medical field is in terms of equity and gaps in professional opportunities. Women face a dizzying barrage of judgements before they open their mouths. One time I was trying to make a proposal about ways in which women should be able to report harassment and threats to their personal safety and careers. Before the meeting, I ran out of my surgery, showered, put on a suit dress, (of course long, which is hard since I am 6'1"), and a suit coat. I did my hair and makeup and made sure I wore nylons. I made sure I didn't look tired or frustrated. I drove across town, walked through hallways covered with male attending pictures, not one woman represented. When I arrived, I was constantly aware of my appearance. I needed to make appropriate eye contact. I had to coach myself to not be either intimidating or intimidated, letting others speak more on any topic.

When offensive comments were made about 'angry women,' making committees. I practiced my box breathing so that I could continue to have a moderately pleasant look on my face. Because of course, I can't be angry or be too opinionated. I can't come off too 'ballsy.' I can't be overly direct. I have to be appropriately thankful for assistance in this arena where they couldn't possibly comprehend the challenges we go through. None of the men at that meeting needed to care about the tone of their voice. How loud their laugh was. If they changed out of scrubs or looked sloppy. They didn't need to worry if they came off as trying too hard. If they were too attractive or unattractive. A million judgements about me and my seriousness as a colleague are made before I opened my mouth.

Of course, the men in that room were 'allies,' - it's even more stressful when dealing with adversaries. With them, you're minimized and demonized before you start talking. You're dramatic or disruptive, too young, inexperienced. Maybe they think they saw some cleavage and comment on how you were trying to be too sexual and attention-seeking.

Perhaps you didn't wear makeup and they get to comment to you that you look tired. 'Maybe you're taking on too much as a mother and physician.' I'm confused as to when motherhood became a truly pre-existing condition to nullify a woman's involvement in change. If you're really lucky, they get to comment about your weight, outfit, hair, and that's so they don't have to listen to a word you say. If on the off chance they hear you, they've given their time, they can quickly talk about how your voice was shrill, you weren't pleasant, you didn't smile enough. Also, you didn't have a good enough sense of humor because well, you didn't laugh enough at their jokes. Or potentially, you laughed too much in a grotesque effort to stroke someone's ego so that maybe you can make changes you need to in order to help the community. Then they get to wonder out loud if your husband is in the picture. They get to decide if you secretly want to have sex with whatever person you were meeting with.

Sadly, most of these details get back to you because there is usually one statistical woman in the room during these discussions and she is close to invisible to them. She could be an assistant, administrator, another physician, front desk staff, or medical assistant. They will not take her seriously, so they openly discuss all these toxic elements in front of her so she can call you and explain how you came off to them. This is in an effort to moderate your actions, and hopefully, in the future, you can wear less perfume, laugh quietly and not make as many points during the discussion.

This is the world of women in medicine. Often, we are better surgeons, physicians, partners and colleagues. Frequently, we have fabulous ideas that could help a practice or system. But instead, we are immediately relocated to another room. In the Ruth Bader Ginsberg movie, RBG is at a work party with her husband. She doesn't fit with the men on the one hand or the women who are all stay-at-home wives. This is where women are in medicine. Somewhere in the middle. We are trying to reach for a brass ring that only continues to rise higher in the air so that some can continue to abuse the power they have.

Since the COVID epidemic started, I have been able to spend more time at home with my son and daughter. I couldn't help but watch them play with clay the other day. It was older, so it wasn't as pliable as it once was. The color wasn't as vibrant. They molded it and bent it and pounded it into whatever shape they wanted it to be. Clay doesn't fight back, and its sole purpose is to exist to make the user happy, to be molded into what they want. I realized I had been the equivalent of clay for way too long. I let myself be pulled, molded, slapped, to try to fit a shape someone else wanted to use. My entire existence was to make my user happy. I tried; I laughed when I was supposed to, I was the first one at work, last one to leave, I worked day in and day out, hoping to have the privilege to continue working. But, clay gets tired of being smacked around. The cracks show in the resistance and it gets hardened. Eventually, it won't do what you want it to do. Ultimately, clay will dry out and be exactly whatever it is meant to be.

Don't forget the game is chess, not poker...

When you go to medical school and residency, you come out wholly ill-prepared to deal with the real world. Yes, you can treat patients. Yes, you have a noble calling and want to put your entire heart into your job. However, you meet people and have to go through things you never dreamed imaginable. I always assumed that, when I became a doctor, everyone would have the same good intentions, put safety first, fight for what was right and just. As women, we have to realize these things are not true. And even worse, it is detrimental for you to believe that everyone will have the same philosophies as you.

I am going to give you some advice I wish I had gotten before I started working. First and foremost, you do you. What does that mean? You run your own professional race. Don't look to the left or to the right. When I started medical school, I hated those jokes about someone failing out. 'Look to the right, look to the left, one of you will be gone by the end of the year.' Stop looking around, only look forward and toward the path you want to go on because, if you keep looking to the side, you are going to run into a tree, and it will be an old, curmudgeon of a tree that casts a huge shadow on your life. Figure out your path and get on it.

Keep the receipts... I mean all of them. If something doesn't feel right to you, save a copy. Send emails from bosses, co-workers, administrators, whoever you don't feel comfortable with, whoever sends you inappropriate information or discussion pieces to your personal accounts. Get all the details in writing. Don't fall into the trappings of some obligatory conversation with someone who will put you down and lie about you. Instead, make sure things are documented. If someone has a problem, get it documented and save a copy. If someone sends you inappropriate texts, save them. If you feel like you can't trust someone, don't. You need to file all these things away, put them in a fireproof safe, because you absolutely need to protect yourself. You worked too hard for too long to make it through this education to have it taken away by someone else. Believe it or not, your intuition can be strong and you need to listen in business, because after all, taking care of patients is a calling, but surviving in the world to work another day is a business.

You control your own narrative. Yes, you do. As hard as it is to see this reality as a new graduate, you need to start building the 'you' that you want to be professionally. Pick pillars in your life that excite you. In my life, I am really passionate about my patients, so patient care is my number one life force; patient and staff safety, writing, journalism, and education. If something doesn't fit into this platform of how I want to live my life, I say no to it. You are going to be too busy to take on every task. You are going to be pulled in a million different directions. You say yes only to the things that fill your life with passion and joy.

This leads me into my next, very important point. You need to be able to say, 'No.' You have to be strong enough to not be guilted by people into doing things you don't want to do. You may just not feel comfortable doing that one favor, meeting that one person for coffee, going to that one event. It doesn't matter what anyone else thinks. Whenever anything professionally doesn't feel right, you say, 'No.' Many people, but especially women, get used and abused by senior staff when they get into practice. They feel that they're paying their dues and will eventually be treated with the same respect as the men at the top of the flagpole. Well, in theory, that could happen; however, it has been the majority of our experiences that you are being used to further another person's agenda, whatever that may be.

No amount of extra work or sacrifice from your family, is going to protect you from whatever tsunami is headed your way. The only people you are responsible for in terms of happiness are yourself and your family. Give yourself the freedom and grace to choose you over anyone else. I always put my job first, tried to be perfect, tried to see the most patients, do the most tasks, be the first person there and last person to leave. You know where that got me? Nowhere. It helped me with nothing in my life. It didn't win any awards for me. It didn't write any articles for me. It didn't help me get involved with teaching health education in high school or helping to make sure Minnesota schools are safe to return after COVID or after the next pandemic that might be plunged into. No, I did that on my own, outside of work. So, follow your passions. They won't lead you astray. Follow your heart because you will often know the truth before your head wants to believe it. For too long, new graduates haven't realized how to win the game. We have to realize we can't bluff our way through life; we need to bring the receipts, pack the punch, and learn how to play chess.

I'm not anyone's sweetheart, young lady, honey or babe… at least at work

My grandfather, whom I loved as much as I could love another human being, doted on us as kids. For the short time we had him in our lives, we knew he loved us in return. He was, as you know, a Lutheran Minister. He was always on call for his parish and was beloved by many. He had a very disarming charm and sense of humor; many would grumble at his corny jokes. One of the things I have taken from him is that how you make people feel is how they remember you. I'll say that again: you have the power to heal and help by making others feel loved and valued. He also had nicknames for us kids. He called my brother, 'tough guy.' He was the only boy in our brood. He called us girls, 'young lady.' To me, because of the way he used that phrase it became synonymous with, 'I love you.' You can of course use this phrase with a variety of tones to express love, excitement, anger, frustration and need for punishment. This phrase never carried any malignancy behind it until I got into my adult life.

When I was in medical school and residency, the programs were academic and traditional and usually very above board in terms of culture. There was one attending who did, however, call me honey and talk about my weight, even in front of those in our care. On this rotation we would do rounds together and go room to room seeing those patients. I would be wearing dress attire and a white coat because some of the specialties and rotations required formality. When you worked with older men, I knew that I had to look particularly well put together. This doctor would often make comments about my hair or lack of makeup. He would tell me that I shouldn't look worse than someone who is post-op. He reminded me that I looked worse than a cancer patient when I didn't wear makeup. All these things seemed like non-issues to me, and at this point I had a fairly-tough skin. I was used to being blamed for wrongdoing of residents when I was a medical student. I was used to being yelled at and sometimes having my hands slapped in the OR. Hell, as a medical student, scrubbed into a case, I stood behind a surgical attending and retracted both superiorly and inferiorly for four hours to provide better visualization. However, what I hated was that he used all my terms of endearment to patronize me. 'Honey, sweetheart, young lady...' It was like nails on a chalkboard.

One day when we were walking into a patient room, he knocked on the door and greeted the patient. She was alert, recovering well and it looked like she was going to leave later that day. He looked at me and made many glib comments to her about my appearance. He discussed endometrial cancer risk factors with the patient, noting that being overweight is a risk factor for cancer. He said, 'Don't be like Dr. Stecher here and let yourself go. It's important to make sure to keep the weight off.'

That definitely made me feel salty. I had been working my butt off, taking pages all night every night. I had worked more than 100 hours that week, and it didn't matter what I did; I was still a thing to be commented on in a room as an overweight woman. He laughed his passive-aggressive laugh. I couldn't tell why he had this animosity towards me, perhaps it is the outward manifestation of his own low self-esteem or inferiority complex. He was part of the only rotation with which I ever struggled.

As I got older, I realized that men used certain 'terms of endearment' to disarm women. When I met different attendings, bosses, administrators, I often started out liking when they called me young lady or hun, honey. It felt like they cared. Well, that's what they do; they disarm you. You are more likely to agree with them and less likely to fight back if you think there is a mutual loyalty and friendship. All this does is render your arguments useless and gives them power over you professionally.

Don't get me wrong; people with whom I have an actual relationship can call me whatever they want. However, men shouldn't be able to use these names in an attempt to minimize us professionally. They shouldn't get more power from putting us in a box off to the side. I am no longer going to be anyone's 'baby' unless you've earned a place in my life and worked for loyalty and trust.

Trapped

There are many times I felt trapped in my life, both personally and professionally. It seemed impossible for me to gain any traction. I felt like I was wading through quicksand. As a physician, I felt completely trapped within my career as soon as I signed my first loan documentation at the beginning of medical school. We had multiple financial seminars detailing how the only physicians who defaulted on their loans were the ones who weren't practicing medicine. To me, this was horrifying. Not only did I need to graduate, I needed to graduate residency and I needed to be in a successful practice that wasn't affected by financial hardships.

There are moments of panic you go through as a young physician. Am I doing the right things? Is this business going to be viable? I had to worry about all these political dynamics that I never imagined I would have needed to consider as a student.

Contracts can trap you so you end up in a precarious financial situation. When we get out of residency, we are naive and believe that all people want the same things in the medical community. Too many people don't completely read their contracts, and don't have a lawyer or mentor review the fine print. To young physicians, I say get a good lawyer! This will pay off over time. I would struggle through my career without the best lawyer in the Twin Cities. However, I may be a little biased. After all, this poor man has had to listen to me for years now. He was on the phone with me when I have gotten bad news, good news, contract negotiations and career planning. There was a moment I was so frustrated that he had to put up with me screaming and crying, little bit of heart break, little bit of being overwhelmed, frustrated and angry to the next level.

We're all going to go through times we feel trapped and we have to decide what we're going to do about it. I have been told so many crazy things in my life to try to kill my spirit. 'You can't do that.' 'Don't go to medical school.' 'You can't afford college, go to the technical schools.' 'You're not cute enough to be on the news.' 'You won't be a good leader.' 'You can't make a difference.' 'You're one person, what can you do? Nothing.' 'There is nothing you can do that is worthwhile.'

In each of those moments I had a decision to make. Each moment ended up being a battle cry for me. There is a switch that flips in my mind, and if you tell me I can't do something, won't do something, can't seek justice or success or do what's right, that basically is like saying 'game on.' To all the people out there feeling trapped. To the people stuck in whatever circumstances in which they feel they are being held hostage. To the people being told 'you can't!' I want you to tell yourself and the people who are hurting you, 'watch me!'

There is no better justice or revenge than propelling yourself into success. Make them watch you grow. Make them see what they did and live to regret how you were treated. They will come to understand that will be remembered and they may well appear, in some form, in a book you write.

Don't Run...

When things get hard in life, our instincts often control our behavior and emotion. When we are confronted with an assault on who we are, what we want, the things we want to accomplish, it is very easy to slip into fight or flight mode. I will tell you, it used to be easier for me to run and hide. I tried to avoid conflict at all costs. I was trained from a young age that conflict got you nowhere in life except into more conflict. I spent the vast majority of my adult life trying to make other people happy so that the tension or conflict in the room would be brought down to a quiet mumble.

However, at some point, I realized that mentality actually acted as a handicap for me in life, relationships, and business. While it is important to be a team player, and make sure others are happy and secure, you should be able to have an opinion and stand your ground without fear of the house of cards falling down around you.

Four years ago, I was trying to get a patient safety issue addressed. I had told a friend how frustrated I was about the response and really wanted to fix the problem. He told me something that helped me get through several hard moments in my career. 'Never Run.' It seems really easy to say, but in fact, it is a painful challenge to live up to those two words.

Living in this mindset, to me, means that you see your

challenges through to the end. If you are trying to do the right and just thing, you show up, and you make sure you don't run away when things get hard. If you're fighting for safety issues for patients, staff, or yourself, you will continue to be persistent and determined in what you're trying to accomplish. In relationships you are there and support your friend or partner no matter what. You show up, you take up space, you work hard, and you don't leave until you've done what you needed to do.

Mom Life...

Any mom knows there is no clock in or out when it comes to your kids. Their health, safety, and happiness pretty much direct everything that you do as a parent. My kids are now five and seven and they still often fall asleep with me. When I was in residency and had my son, every night when I got home, I would feed him and snuggle him until he fell asleep. Then I would put him into his bassinet or crib. This became what I did with him every day of his life. When my daughter was born, we carried on the tradition and both of them would fall asleep with me.

As a working, first-time, new mom, I felt guilty about everything. I remember when I was driving into an overnight call during my second trimester, I started crying because I really had no idea how I was going to be productive, a good physician, and mom. I worried about being present for my kids. I worried about what kind of mom I would be. I worried there was some pre-programming that happened in my brain and I wouldn't be able to be what they needed.

Every mom has a different style of parenting. I am the hugging, smooching, telling my kids I love them 100 times a day mom. And that is right for me. What I tell my patients when they confide in me their concerns are that you have to find your own way. What is right for me isn't right for the next person. You have to run your own race in this marathon of parenthood. If breastfeeding works for you, great; if it doesn't it's ok. If you are able to stay home with your kids all the time, and that fulfills you, great. If you can't do it or want to go to work, also equally great.

Does there have to be compromise? Of course, your children come first but it doesn't mean you sacrifice the rest of your life, you just have to work out how to make it all come together. While you may think you are the first to struggle with the tightrope between parenthood and career, you are not, nor will you be the last. It is called life. The good news is that we can learn from those that came before us.

Mom shaming is an unfortunate part of our culture right now. I had hoped that COVID 19 would help people develop more grace for others; however, I have often found this to be the opposite. In Minnesota we had our first COVID case in early March and you could see the divisions start almost immediately. There were people who didn't believe COVID would affect us, or it would have a predilection to individuals with different ethnic backgrounds. As someone in science, this was very bothersome to me.

We started seeing moms on both sides of the COVID battle shaming moms on the other side of the fight. There were those who dutifully wore the masks and there were the anti-maskers. Never in my wildest imagination could I have predicted the different scenarios I have seen play out at parks with kids listening. I could never have dreamed that a virus that is affecting people of all ethnicities, ages, and locations could lead to a political turf war. This is unconscionable in my opinion.

As the seasons changed to talk of fall and school, the mom shaming amped up its game. It seemed everyone developed more and more polarized views on school and what is safe. To me, the choices should be grounded in data, research, and what has worked in other countries. It should not be based on news soundbites or media headlines. You have children, you have a duty to put some effort into digging deep and researching all available material that will help toward an informed decision. However, it has turned into one political party accusing another of dramatizing the concern to control elections with vested interests driving the narrative instead of us rationally listening to experts in science and medicine, many of whom appear to have had their careers curtailed for simply questioning the direction of travel or asking if we have explored all opportunity of care.

I have seen moms yell at other moms 'dumb,' 'unable to have original thought,' and 'brainwashed!' for not letting their kids go back to school full-time or part-time. I would like to think that we can all unite as moms and acknowledge, 'My job is to protect my kids and their safety and happiness to the best I can.' For you those decisions may look different than for me. If we are all trying to do the right things, I don't know why this is even an argument. Regardless of which side of any debate we may be, if we put our heads together we stand a much better chance to arrive at the right conclusion while conserving our strength for the real battles in life.

Quest for Connection

My daughter and son sat staring at each other on the park grass. They started yelling something. I couldn't quite make it out at first.

'You're more beautiful!'

'You're more handsome!'

'No, you're more beautiful.'

'No, you're more handsome.'

While they were screaming at each other, they were throwing grass clippings and laughing. Addie then jumped on JJ and started tickling him until they ran off to swing on the swing set together. Their laughter was so genuine and pure. They are completely open and authentic with each other and don't hide behind a mask of who they want to portray. They aren't worried about an image or propaganda to sell to the world and are vulnerable and real. Why does that ever stop? Why can't people be who they are or who they are supposed to be without fear of their insecurities being weaponized against them?

It's been my experience that most people become like paintings in need of restoration. People are weathered, they are hardened, they are filled with relationships that hurt them, and inauthenticity. However, at the base, underneath all the damage and layers of dirt, the true, genuine, authentic masterpiece is still present.

The Sistine chapel restoration and conservation was one of the most detailed projects of its kind. This project was painstaking and required a labor of love. The experimentation for the project was done in 1979, initial renovations 1980-1984, and the ceiling 1989. After the ceiling, The Last Judgment, a fresco by Michelangelo, was revitalized. These initial parts were presented to the Pope in 1994. The renovation and conservation project then culminated in 1999.

As the restoration artists performed their skilled work, they had many goals: use materials that were proven safe, analyze the art and learn from the great artists, remove the 're-painting' from previous restorers, and remove 500 years of grime, candle deposits, and discoloration. They also worked to conserve surfaces that were in danger of total destruction. These artists and lovers of life also worked to maintain the integrity of the art and preserve the small details.

Now, you may be wondering why on earth art restoration is fascinating to me. Besides having a desperate desire to travel, which I haven't had the chance to because of my many years of education and work, I feel like each one of us is like the Sistine Chapel. We are beautiful, whole, and unique. Our nose, smile, eyes, and laughter lines are some of the fine the details. Our love for each other brings the color out in the frescos. Our empathy and humanity can light up the ceiling that drapes over the chapel.

Everyone in our lives changes the structure and detail. Each person has the ability to act as a skilled artist, willing to accentuate our history. However, frequently there are restorers with no experience, who can blur the lines, ruining the art work. The people we come into contact with can blow out the candles too close to the fresco and cover it with soot and dust, acting to deteriorate the colors we worked so hard to show the world.

The further in life we get and the more abuse the painting takes, it makes it nearly impossible for people to see what is behind the dirt and destruction. It's easier to dehumanize someone if we are living in dirt and rubble ourselves. It's easy to look at a person and only see the layer of filth that has accumulated over the years.

I've found that loving someone helps bring out the vibrance of your fresco as well as theirs. The colors tend to illuminate not only yourself, but others around you. You can pay attention to the details and wash off the grime. You can look in your heart and repair the ceiling. By doing this, hopefully, the vibrance of your architecture can shine enough light so others can work on their own Sistine Chapels. The vibrance of your love and kindness can be magnified if you are in the right museum. My best advice is to be authentically you and stay away from the people who walk too close blowing out candles.

One Fine Day...

You ever just have a day where you feel broken? More broken then usual? You end up getting onto a bobsled from hell, and you spiral south with every second. Since COVID, many of my days could be characterized as a roller coaster. I was watching the movie Sabrina, with Harrison Ford, a few weeks ago. I loved this movie as a kid; however, now I definitely feel like I have been Sabrina a time or two in my life. This poor girl with low self-confidence, goes away, finds herself, and some jerky guy uses her to accomplish what he wants. It is a tale as old as time. Anyway, during the movie the line, 'Only living organ donor,' is used when describing one of the characters. It is meant as a negative because he, of course, is a crabby, business-focused, egocentric character. However, I think this could apply to me, or any mom, healthcare worker, or hard-working person on earth right now.

I went through my life trying to keep people at a distance. I seemed like an open book to many, however, I never really gave people the inside track to be able to hurt me. I was solely focused on what I needed to do in life. There isn't a lot of room for extraneous things when you are caught up in your job.

I had this moment the other day, when I was talking to my partner, who is also a mom, where I think we were both just done with everything. My day had started at 11:30 pm the night before, technically, as I drove back into the hospital for a delivery. I did a vaginal delivery at 12:00 on the nose. During a delivery you are constantly aware of a multitude of factors. You are analyzing every data point on a continual and simultaneous basis. How are they pushing? How is the pain control? What is the position of the baby? Is she on Pitocin? Has she had a fever? How does the baby look on the monitor? Did she have her two doses or more of antibiotics if her GBS was positive? As the pushing progresses you watch for more data. Is the baby still tolerating the process? Do we have the tools we need? If the heart tones go down, is she going to want a section or vacuum delivery? Is she close enough for a vacuum delivery? What was her last ultrasound? Is the baby too big for her? Do I have to worry about a shoulder dystocia? Is she having blood sugar issues?

Then they turn a corner and all of a sudden, they may have bleeding. You think… is it bleeding from a tear? How are her tissues? How swollen is she? Is she still making progress? I hope she can have a vaginal delivery. She may need repair vaginally, even with a section, if bleeding. Does the baby still look good? More bleeding could mean abruption? As the head crowns and you coach your patient to make sure she is effectively pushing, you ready the table so you can grab the tools easily. Clamp, scissors, bulb suction, ring forceps in case the placenta is hard to get out.

As the baby's head emerges, there is always the moment where you are delivering the shoulders of the baby that, as an OBGYN, you are thinking, if there is a shoulder dystocia, does she have space, what would work to get the baby out safely? Once the baby is out and on the mom's chest, you go to work on the placenta. Some people will easily let the placenta deliver. Some people will have bleeding and you need to massage their uterus more aggressively to remove it. Some people will have retained placentas, and if they have an epidural, it is much easier to help them guide this out. After placenta delivers you are always looking for sources of bleeding. Is the uterus contracting? Is the tone good? Does she need medication to help with bleeding? Does she have a tear? Does she have a new infection in the uterus?

All the bleeding investigation happens instantaneously in your mind. You are feeling, looking, watching the rate, making orders for medication, repairing tears as you work. When you're finished, you walk out of the room and go to the next activity. By this point on that particular day, it was only 12:30 am. You then repeat that process three to seven more times, sometimes doing a cesarean section or several more deliveries. Sometimes you have other gynecological emergencies as well, surgeries you need to perform, dilation and curettage for bleeding, maybe someone has an ovarian cyst that has ruptured or an ovarian torsion. Potentially you have someone roll into the ER with a ruptured ectopic pregnancy, you need to emergently take her to the operating room to save her life, and all the while thinking about the blood products, transfusion protocol, and surgical needs.

All physicians are then hit with a constant stream of patient questions and messages while dealing with emergencies. I've been called at 2 a.m. during a ruptured ectopic to talk about a persistent yeast infection for two weeks. In the middle of the night, I have been called about a headache in a non-pregnant person that goes away with Tylenol but is annoying and has been present for four days while I am actively trying to save someone's life. I fully anticipate this and understand the need, however, when you don't hear back in five to ten minutes, please realize we may be trying to deal with an emergency.

By the time you run into clinic the next morning, you have been up for more than twenty-four hours, and you were managing your patients overnight. You look at the schedule, see many patients with many needs, many procedures. You look at your inbox with more than twenty patient calls. You have to review lab reports for twenty to forty patients. Patients message you questions to respond to as well, all while you're trying to answer pages, stay on schedule, dealing with unexpected emergencies and miscarriages and grief. Patients are struggling with COVID, and the stress is genuine. That makes their mental health a real concern to be dealt with during this process. However, that means you are falling behind, and then people start to get angry that you are delayed.

Almost like clockwork on a busy day, you will be called to the hospital for an additional emergency or delivery. On this day, I had a hemorrhage to deal with. I ran across the hall to the hospital. Again, you are taking in a million data points. What was her last Hgb? Has she had any high blood pressures? This could mean she has pre-eclampsia, which can affect platelets. Does she have a bleeding history or a coagulopathy? These answers would change the approach. Did she deliver easily? Have any tears? Did your partner think they got the placenta out completely? Could she have retained products? Does she have tone? Is her IV working? Do we need another IV? You simultaneously gather data and give orders, Methergine, Hemabate, Cytotec, TXA, open Pitocin, get her labs, cbc, type and cross, PT, INR PTT, Fibrinogen, CMP if she is hypertensive .

You put your hand inside of the patient's uterus to slow the bleeding and determine whether the uterine tone is appropriate or if you can feel anything abnormal. Does she have a uterine inversion? Should we open the operating room? Is the rate slowing? Once everything is taken care of, you march quickly back to the clinic and pick up where you left off, trying to not look tired, and maintain a smile, because if you don't, then you're labeled difficult or crabby.

Once you're back, you realized all the morning patients who were canceled have just been added onto the afternoon. You are double-booked with new patients. You have unexpected procedures. You have to make sure to wear your mask and your shield at all times. You find out a person you delivered may have had COVID during delivery. You try to provide excellent care to everyone. Then the messages keep coming from every angle, the pages don't stop, you're trying to stay on time, and make as few people upset as possible.

Then a scheduler comes to yell at you and proclaim, 'I told you when you do the affirmation. It has to be done this way.'

'Ok. I will do it when I have time. Is it needed now?'

'No, she isn't seeing it now.'

'Ok. I will do it when I have time.'

The epic notes come: can you add this order, can you

put this in, can you order these labs for tomorrow? Can this person get an order for this lab in a week and ultrasound put in today? The breast center called; the radiologist wants an order for an ultrasound. Can you add that now?

You feel like all the little things, charting, orders, administrators not understanding, all of it is falling on your shoulders and you are essentially drowning with no help and no ability to continue in a timely fashion. You get transfers and you don't have all the patient records and are trying to piece things together to not miss something. You take care of infertility patients who have been seen at four locations and need to follow the cycles, all along feeling like you aren't valued, appreciated, or helped. Likely, you are being told you aren't working fast enough, and you can't have an opinion on how things are run. If you're really lucky, you'll have someone who is COVID positive slip through the screening and be a new patient sitting in a room, for a non-urgent reason, exposing your staff. And what is COVID positive when the main test has already been shown to be wildly inaccurate?

You then send someone else over to labor and delivery for new blood pressure issues. The decision you make is to start induction. All you want is to sleep, rest, turn off your brain, and not worry about something work related. You sign out at what time? now having been up for two days. You go home, take care of the kids, get them ready for bed.

My five-year-old year old always gets upset if I can't snuggle her until she falls asleep, so, both of my kids fall asleep on me while I read the latest research articles about COVID, returning to school, and planning for the next couple months. Since my kids are remote learning, I have to look at the meetings planned for that over the next day or two. You realize family and friends have messaged you, but you're too tired to respond. Maybe one day I can be invested again in something other than work.

The kids are then put in their beds, I sit back down and read another article. By then it is WHAT TIME? 23:00. I go to sleep, wake up five hours later, and start the process over again. It's hard because I often feel pulled in a million directions. Usually, I love being needed and feeling useful, but lately it has felt extra taxing. Like no other time before, I have been depleted by my job and not sustained by it. COVID has made every interaction a little more challenging and requires a little more energy to be expended .

Grief...

When you have a collision between being overworked and grief, you can feel like you've dug yourself a grave. I read my kids a book about filling other people's buckets. Yes, this seems immature, but it's really important. People either take from us, give to us, or both. We can choose to be people who go out of our way to support others. This in turn fills their proverbial 'emotional bucket.' If we take from them, we are essentially depleting their ability to cope with the world.

Lately again, because of COVID, I have felt like my bucket has been more depleted at baseline. There are a lot of extra stresses and concerns that go with working in healthcare. This, unfortunately, is why we need to find our people. The people we love can help us restore to a state that is as normal as we can exist in at this time.

What happens when you get a collision between grief and this depletion? Well, you get what many of us in healthcare are going through right now. We are running on a near empty tank of gas, which we all know you can't do in Minnesota winters. Otherwise, the gas tank freezes up and you stall, ending up stuck in a snow bank. Not that I am speaking from experience, but somehow, we need to fill each other up and give each other grace.

Many healthcare workers feel a sense of moral injury

now. We are all going through grief on a small scale, just missing when life was easier to navigate. Doctors still take a Hippocratic oath to do no harm, and if you're like me, that extends to staff, partners and patients. If you extrapolate that out, you feel a moral responsibility to protect them and keep them safe.

There are many guidelines, including governmental, that have been put in place to manage the pandemic. Some seem to go against the way physicians work. If our life's work is to protect people, it's hard to go into situations where we aren't equipped to deal with that task. This creates frustration and grief for some. It hurts our ability to trust and have faith in the system. In many places, physicians have felt they've been hung out to dry and treated as if they're replaceable. After all, for much of my career I had someone continually telling me I was replaceable, so it's not a far jump to get to that thought process.

To you I want to stress that you aren't replaceable, you aren't expendable, you are as perfect and as imperfect as you are by varying degrees at any one time. We all need to feel valued and loved and supported, and if no one else supports you, I will.

When coping mechanisms honed over a lifetime get depleted, it also becomes harder to manage grief. Things tend to bubble up in our own lives. We lose the ability to compartmentalize what we had done successfully before.

We all go through losses in life. Some of these losses are huge, dramatic, chaotic, life changing events. We lose children, partners, loved ones, friends, jobs. Some of us go through traumas and feel betrayed by ourselves or another person. When you have been through a trauma or hurt beyond normal abilities to comprehend, you also grieve for the life you had. You grieve for the person you were before the seminal event happened.

Grief enters our lives in many ways. It usually moves in with no intent of leaving. It simply pours a new foundation, picks out siding, and becomes our home. Grief can become an adversarial neighbor when your usual weapons against these interferences become worthless. Now, some of us accept grief initially, almost as if we've invited it into our lives. Sometimes, we feel like we deserve the grief, blame ourselves for whatever happened, and we take it on as a constant companion.

The problem is when we have decided this new neighbor has worn out its welcome. Grief can then become deceptive. Some days become good and manageable and some cast a looming shadow on everything we do. There are moments when you become so desperate for the sun you can't imagine living in the storm any longer. You start to question purpose. You question people and their place in your life. You wonder what was real or if you surrounded yourself with fake individuals throughout your life.

Grief then can hide in us. People who really care can see it in our eyes. It tends to hang out in the corners of our heart where love once existed for a person from the past. The places where joy, happiness, and fun took up residence are now filled with this ominous predator. People in our lives that don't know the truth of our world will often make comments about our process. 'Suck it up.' 'Move on.' 'We've moved on, why haven't you?' There is nothing more triggering to someone going through a major life event than telling them how you've moved on and wondering why she or he can't. Most individuals would love to move on. They are in fact, at this moment, angry at themselves that they are hurting. They want to be back to normal. However, they don't get to decide when this is done, and I would argue it's going to be with them in some degree for the rest of their lives.

Some people are better equipped to manage these emotions. Some are able to compartmentalize, put it in a box, slide it to the top of the closet, and shut the door. Others, who are more like me, think it's sealed and then different events will trigger the opening of the box and throw the debris in our faces. People's smells, cologne, the sound of their footsteps, or a song, can elicit a grief response. It's unfortunate that my memory is as good as it is because all the good and the bad is frozen in time for me to play on the reruns.

One of my patients asked me if I had ever had my heart broken. She was struggling with some major life changes and needed to talk to someone. During COVID, our normal social circles have broken down, and often we feel more alone when dealing with these matters. I smiled and looked at her. She obviously just needed to feel like someone understood what she was going through. I said, 'Of course, if you have the ability to actual love someone, then everyone gets their heart broken.'

She then asked me, 'How did you get over it?'

Well, in that moment I had two choices, tell her the truth, or tell her that I got over it. I told her I never really got over it. It's something I carry with me, like a shadow. Some days I don't notice the feelings. Some days are empirically hard. However over time, you feel the pain less. You start being able to remember the good associated with a person. Some of the space fills back up with happiness and joy. The weight of it becomes easier to carry.

I was trying to explain grief to a friend who hasn't had any real hardship or loss in his life. He's a perfect surgeon who had always been the dumper and not the one dumped upon. His parents are blissfully happy and he lives in the sunshine. I used my best medical analogy to paint the picture for him.

Grief to me, is like a giant wound infection. Sometimes the infection is so bad it gets into your blood stream and you become septic. You need medical attention. You can get admitted to the ICU on life support. You can need surgery and IV antibiotics. You end up feeling as if you're never going to get better and you are always going to be critically ill. Over time, the infection gets cleared out of your blood stream, you start breathing off the ventilator.

The antibiotics assist with the wound itself. You then meet criteria for a wound vac. This is placed over the hole that resides in your flesh. The entire purpose is to make this hole smaller. This process is painful. You need to look at this hole and change your own dressings to make sure you're healing. Eventually, the vac is removed and now you are on to regular dressing changes. You live in a semi constant fear that you will get infected again, that the same issues are going to crop up in your life.

You start to wonder about the infection. Why? Why did

this happen? Why wasn't I able to fight the infection? Did I do something wrong? I tried really hard to be perfect. How can I prevent this from happening again? How can I make sure to never go through this pain again? And there are usually no answers.

Most of the time we recover. In some cases, you are left with small defects in your tissue. If the infection threatened your life, you may end up with some permanent health issues. You heal the best you can and then try to put one foot in front of the other to move on.

Purgatory

When I was in college, I was part of a program called Lasallian Honors at St. Mary's University of Minnesota. This program was geared toward developing students into servant leaders who put the community and safety of others ahead of all else. I actually loved this program because it fit with my core beliefs. These principles are what guide my life and how I practice medicine.

Like most college students, we read Dante's Inferno. Purgatory is the second part of Dante's Divine Comedy. We discussed that this mystical location resides somewhere between heaven and hell. In the poem it is a mountain in the Southern Hemisphere. In Dante's vision, there are multiple segments; bottom section (ante-purgatory) which is made of seven levels of suffering and spiritual growth. Interestingly, this segment consists of pride, envy, wrath, sloth, extreme greed for wealth or material gain, excessive or extravagant spending, gluttony and lust. The souls in purgatory are thought to be suffering not only to pay a debt to God, as many philosophers like Thomas Aquinas depicted, but also to be enlightened and transformed. Theologians hypothesized the evolution of your soul could take thousands of years.

There is a park by my house and across from one of my current and past clinics named Purgatory Park. I used to go there during my lunch hour in what seems like a previous life. Somehow the name seems cryptically fitting. I have gone to this park more times than I can count. I would often walk around the water to get clarity on the day. Sometimes I would have lunch with a friend. We would talk about nothing and everything. It only seems fitting that my soul would go to commune with other seemingly lost souls.

Over the last couple of years, I have had many conversations in purgatory, some horrible, heartbreaking, anxiety provoking, enraging, light-hearted, happy and hopeful. I have now often taken my children there to walk around the water. As I have gotten stronger through life, I have climbed up the mountain, and being there now brings me less pain. However, I think the theologians were right; we are trapped in purgatory, until we learn about ourselves, our past mistakes, and the people who reside with us.

Many of us land in purgatory because of love. We are left with the layers of suffering that comes with mismanaging the most important part of being human. However, love is the only entity strong enough to pull us from hell or purgatory and land us in paradise. When I think about the state of the world now amidst COVID, if we could be more virtuous in our love for each other; we would be able to climb this mountain and make it through the hell we created on earth. We all need to walk the path through the inferno alongside Dante. It's the only thing that will help us make it through the current crisis of culture .

The Villain or the Hero?

There are countless times I wish the villains would have revealed themselves before I became entangled in the narrative. I have often felt like I was living in a Greek tragedy. It's easy to get engulfed in a situation with a tragic hero, which Aristotle would define as a man who is virtuous but not 'eminently good.' These men always seem good, moral, hardworking, but often find themselves in a fortune reversal because of an ingrained flaw. A shortcoming they have as a person that they can't admit to and won't work through. Their inability to accept the truth often leads down a journey of darkness and destruction for anyone who knows and loves them.

Sadly, many of us, have 'hamartia,' a tragic flaw in life. We can either go on a road to discover this flaw and correct it or we can stay stagnant and struggle with alcohol addiction, weight issues, multiple disruptive love relationships, or any other destructive behaviors. As physicians, we all try to help our patients live their best lives. We try to offer assistance to get them on a path to recovery, whether it is from mental or physical suffering. The hardest part I have found is having people in your life you can't help break out of their flawed existence.

At times we face course changing moments. Some moments are so powerful that you are able to watch them from outside yourself. They destroy who you once were and a new person is able to emerge. You become aware that the wounds are too deep for a once naive heart to survive. You absorb every second of the event and can remember the details as if you're standing in the room, silently watching your life's destruction.

I lived my life putting up walls. Each had a slightly different proximity to my core. Each person existed in a different orbit. I was fully prepared for most people coming in and out of my life. Some would be like shooting stars, we would have a great run, and then the light would go out. The problem for me has always been the people who sneak their way in. They seemingly earn a relationship. They're present day in and day out, working to earn trust. They become who you turn to in times of good and bad. These people are complex entities. You're not prepared for them. They catch you off balance. They act as if they already have the keys to your life because somehow, they do. These are the people who promise to be there, that they wouldn't hurt you, and that they aren't going anywhere. Somehow, over time the walls get broken down, only to reveal that they should have stayed up, and in fact been reinforced.

I have only been truly broken once, and it's when I accidentally let someone into every chapter of my life and then needed to quickly erase that person from time. It was as if I lived with a ghost by my side who could come and go. It's important to remember that these people are part of the story for a reason. They teach you to not externalize anything that you can give yourself, like your power. Once a man or woman has power over how you perceive yourself, all is lost. You are hostage to the other person's moods, whims and desires.

I have found it stunning how these people can sneak into your life. At times I have felt as if I am looking at a person through a reflection in glass. In that moment you could be going on with your life, and look up, and there is the person, staring at you through the scrub cabinet door. The person seems so real and present, but you can't touch him or her. You end up wondering if anything was more real than the simple reflection. This is true in many relationships; you can be at a loss for what was real and what was pretend. However, some people have an intrinsic capability of making you wonder if the entire thing was a mirage like the reflection. It's important to accept that these people don't know how to be any more present than that glass. Often, they don't live life with enough color to exist in the three-dimensional world. It's up to you to understand that you are going to live with all the vibrancy life has to offer.

Instead of falling to the ghosts, you need to find value in knowing you are capable of true, honest, wanting nothing in return, do-anything love. I used to ask myself, 'Why wasn't I worth it?' 'What did I do?' 'What could I change to be worthy?' 'How can I belong?' I spent my entire life trying to find my place to be. When I thought I had, it went to ash before my eyes. I realized I was asking the wrong person for answers. All the time, I should have been directing them at myself. I had given my power away for so long I didn't know it was there.

You can give yourself love and a place to belong. You are everything you need. Finding a partner in life, friendships and work environment are all nice things to have. However, until you can find yourself and your place in the scheme of things, then you are going to be trying to fill an endless void through putting expectations on other people that are unlikely to be fulfilled.

Let's talk about sex...

The long and the short of it is... no pun intended... love is not sex and sex is not love. Yes, they can co-exist. However, I have listened to many painful stories my patients have shared where this wasn't clear to them. Culturally, women have been at a disadvantage when it comes to their sex lives. The vast majority of women have grown up with an understanding that sex is bad, you need to wait until marriage, and it is something that shouldn't be discussed.

When I was five-years-old, I was laying on the carpet in front of our television set. My mother was behind me on the couch. This is, of course, during a time when you watched real time television and would go to the scrolling television guide to see what was on currently. She put the TV guide up on the screen. I watched the programs dance by and tried to read all the headings. I was learning to read and treated this as a game. How many could I read before the screen shifted? One title caught my eye, I had heard the word before, but never saw it in print.

'Mom, what is sex? What does sex mean?'

'Nothing Kellie, don't ask silly questions.'

'Mom, what does it mean?'

'Why don't you go play in your room.'

And just as quickly as the word traveled across my vision, the shame associated with the word was also created.

Women, unfortunately, are often made to feel like their sexuality takes a back seat to a male partner's. In many cultures it is still unacceptable for women to enjoy sex or want sex as much as or more than men.

We all hear how relationships are often fraught with mismatched sexual desire. Sometimes guilt, shame, culture, and religion play roles in a woman's desire to have sex.

In countries around the world, we still see women imprisoned or abused for having sex. Female genital mutilation still occurs. I have personally taken care of many patients who have had this procedure done and it serves no beneficial purpose for the girl. It is done to perpetuate cultural norms where a woman needs to remain a virgin until marriage, and her sexual satisfaction is completely discredited. Many believe genital mutilation will keep a woman faithful to her husband. However, women experience many complications from this procedure: chronic pain, infection, fistulas, bladder issues, difficulty with tearing in childbirth, sometimes difficulty having sex with any partner, bleeding, and even death.

If you have been raised in any country where sex is considered taboo, you will likely have difficulty communicating about this topic in future relationships. Many have also been indoctrinated that you can only have sex once married. News flash: patients can't shut off that guilt or shame once they are married. They feel like they are committing an immoral act. This leads to decreased sexual satisfaction, frustration, and sometimes physical pain. If a woman is not able to relax, she can often have pain with sex because of pelvic floor or muscular issues. She may also have decreased lubrication. It's important to realize that women are struggling with these issues, even after marriage.

When women aren't taken seriously as people who can also enjoy sex, they are often embarrassed to talk about sexual functioning. I have met many adult women who have had more than one partner who have never experienced an orgasm. They felt shame and guilt and unable to make any attempt at exploring their sexuality with their partners. They also felt uncomfortable or unwilling to talk about anything intimate with their partner.

The arousal response in women can be complex, and they can make choices about their bodies just like men can. Women can also have sex for a variety of reasons: to have fun, feel better about themselves, feel connected to someone else, conception, because they're in love or they want to make a partner happy. We can't discredit other people's interests and make them feel guilty for having them. We need to stop using sexuality as a tool to create division between the genders. I think that some of the gender equity issues we have globally and in this country stem from how women's sexual health is dealt with and the biases people have toward women and their sexual functioning.

Everyone needs to find a partner in life where they can be completely vulnerable and communicate what they need and want from their sexual experiences. If you don't have someone with whom you can talk candidly about these issues, you need to start having honest conversations with your partner so you and he or she feel comfortable. If you need help or you have questions about pain or emotional concerns you have, please talk to your OBGYN. We are here to help you get through any issues because we want you to live a healthy and fulfilling life in all aspects.

Helmets, seat belts, and parachutes…

I was driving to the hospital for a delivery. Before I left my driveway, I made sure my seatbelt was fastened. Occasionally in the past, I had driven from the hospital physician parking spots to the physician parking structure without my seat belt on. This week when I tried that, I felt guilty and immediately strapped in.

That day when I was turning onto the highway, I saw a 40-something-year-old man on a motorcycle, not wearing a helmet. He was dodging around cars and took the shoulder to get by others. I watched him cut off a car, making the driver swerve as he cut across to exit.

Suddenly, human nature made a little more sense. I was worried about my safety, getting to the hospital to care for a patient, and safely returning home to my kids. This man didn't even care enough about himself to wear a helmet that would potentially prevent him from dying on the side of the road. If he wasn't going to protect himself, why would I think he would protect others? He isn't going to abide by any rules. Rather, he will cut people off, weave in and out, and not think twice about any destruction or chaos he leaves in his wake. If he can't wear a helmet, his risk taking will extend way beyond that.

I totally started questioning safety equipment in general at that point. If people don't care about their own safety or that of their children and community, why do we invest in safety infrastructures? Why don't we just say, 'Here's a seat belt; we know it will protect you in the event of a car crash, but your call.' Maybe when we go sky-diving we could make it like Russian Roulette. Every tenth pack doesn't have a parachute. If you live, you live; if you die, you die. What would be the difference?

If we are going to care about the sanctity of life, then we need to care about all lives. We don't get to pick and choose what we do to help people. We don't get to provide medical care for only those who think like us, and act like us, or look like us. Every life we have the honor of caring for we do with 100% commitment to keep the person healthy. I guess if you don't feel that way, maybe don't wear the belt and don't put the parachute in the pack.

COVID 19

There are moments in life that transcend our collective consciousnesses. COVID has changed how we shop, educate, take care of children, work, run the economy, find love, relate to friends, and view the future. But for those of us in healthcare, it has been a tsunami. Most of us lived in areas that weren't hit hard by the virus immediately, so we were left in preparation mode. We were sitting ducks waiting for the boom to be lowered. We planned, researched, read studies every waking moment of every single day. We prepared ourselves the best we could with the information provided for what we viewed was inevitable.

The doctors, nurses, techs, laboratory and pathology processors, environmental services, and everyone else in healthcare has felt the shocks and aftershocks of preparation. So many in healthcare have been punished for speaking out against policies. Many physicians have had their salaries cut or lost because of the economic impacts of stopping elective surgeries. There are monumental fallouts that everyone has faced. Doctors and nurses have struggled with childcare throughout the pandemic.

When my husband was in quarantine because of possible exposure to COVID, that we couldn't test for because we experienced this during the time when testing was not possible. My sister and her husband would come sit on the deck in our backyard and Facetime with the kids. There were days when everyone took a Facetime shift while they worked on remote learning. I worked sixty plus hours to see patients, do deliveries, emergency surgeries, take calls and make sure that I was learning everything I could to better serve our community.

What has been liberating about this is the finality of death. As odd as it is to say, COVID has helped me lose whatever fear I had held on to. When COVID reached Minnesota, I was finally starting to get my feet back under me. I had changed jobs and had a tough year in transition. In March I thought that things were finally starting to settle down for the first time in a long time. I was beginning to get used to my new life. I was appreciative of the new people and opportunities that I was given. I loved being part of a more academic system where I could be more involved in education.

I have always been a passionate person. I root for the underdog and I would have David's back against the Goliath. I am unapologetically on a quest to do right by people, and to seek justice for them. When I changed jobs, I thought the new position was a golden opportunity to work on the culture of medicine. Too many women have experienced harassment, physical/sexual assault, intimidation, and threats in terms of their career or family life. Many of our trainees don't have the support they need to come forward. Most women who experience gross abuse of power in the workplace are afraid to come forward out of fear of retaliation. Instead, these women quit medicine altogether, become depressed, some commit suicide, some take on alternate careers like journalism, open new businesses, etc. This is because we appear to be incapable of policing ourselves.

The primary reason I entered into my proposals for cultural change was the fact that I didn't want anyone out in the world feeling as if they were floating on a raft alone or hanging off a cliff on the verge of letting go. I knew what it felt like to be alone, no one to call, and no one to have your back. I knew what a dark place it takes you to when you aren't believed and treated as disposable. I didn't want anyone to face these moments alone.

In that context I viewed cultural changes as a staff and physician safety issue. I started working my way through the administrative hurdles that are part of academic and institutional medicine. I wanted to produce changes whereby we had a reporting system that people could turn to and be taken seriously without fear of retaliation. I wanted to develop support groups so people didn't feel alone. I wanted to have a zero-tolerance policy for people who threatened others in the workplace. The most ambitious change I wanted to make was developing a committee to evaluate allegations, take them seriously, and provide assistance for employees who needed help. During this process I had met or interacted with so many people in the system. It felt like we were getting some traction with this endeavor when COVID hit.

The world stopped. We became part of an alternate reality, one I really didn't care for. The healthcare world was going to respond to this healthcare crisis. We immediately made modifications to schedules in order to try to protect each other. If one of us was going to get ill, we couldn't have the entire group out. Babies want to be born when they want to be born. Patients need healthcare, and emergencies are things we still can't plan for. I, along with one of my partners, read everything remotely related to the knowledge we might need. I joined local and international COVID groups. I networked with national and international OBGYNs.

Somewhere between fighting for equity and trying to protect our patients and staff from COVID, I grew up. I somehow became unafraid. When you become a woman who knows what she wants and makes a plan of how she's going to get it, the rest of it doesn't matter. My focus shifted to safety and advocacy and social justice. I started becoming the person I always wanted to be, the one who was always in my heart, but never allowed to come out.

Every day suddenly provided a valuable reason for pushing the agenda forward. How were we going to make this new world acceptable and safe for all of us? In that moment when I felt like I was getting it together, George Floyd was murdered. Being a physician in the twin cities and having that happen miles from my home rocked our midwestern facade. I realized that the Potemkin village we existed in was far more detailed then even I had comprehended before. Every time I have been frustrated with the world, the country, or our state, I have to stop myself and put it all in perspective.

There are moments when I feel like my work is inconsequential and worthless during the monumental failings around us. Whenever I feel pulled to quit, I usually receive an email or call from a woman, colleague, co-worker, telling me what happened to them in the midst of the pandemic or in terms of gender or racial equity concerns. Every time I am ready to quit, someone reaches out and has given me a new platform because they read something I wrote or said, heard me talk, read a proposal, and I realize what I am doing is having an impact, and if it only helps one person, I will consider myself a lucky human being. You see, I have learned that hope without action is worthless. In order to survive to make a difference you need to own your truth and you need to act in ways that will bring change.

When I was in medical school, we lost power before one of my pharmaceutical tests. This is a class I loved because it was rote memorization and I have a nearly photographic memory. I had an almost perfect score on all the tests. I went through my flashcards using a candle for light. I went to bed early so I could be prepared for my test the next day. As I was getting ready in the morning, I realized we still didn't have power. Then there was an odd, foul smell, that was suspiciously like the odor of tinfoil burning in a microwave, which yes, I did in childhood while babysitting my siblings.

As I was brushing my teeth, I saw firefighters running up to the back porch door. They asked us what we were doing. I said getting ready for school of course. This was the first sign I had that there had been a problem. It turns out our apartment building had an electrical fire. The newspapers said every inhabitant had successfully been evacuated. Well, I was a resident and I slept through the night while the other side of the building was on fire. They said we needed to be removed immediately. I grabbed my bag, my phone, and went to my test, on which I got 100%.

In life, at some point, we are all going to be in the 'fire'. We are going to have choices about how we respond to those fires. COVID is just one of many infernos I have been through and will go through. Each of these situations is a test; each can help you grow or can break you apart. The most beautiful thing about being human is we get to decide the ending to our own stories. We get to decide which direction we go, what we take with us from the fire, and how we do on the tests.

It's up to us to figure out what matters and brings us joy. For me, it's always been love and hope to produce changes we need in the community. My joy has always been working with my patients and getting to deliver babies, helping patients with their surgery, and being there for them when times are hard. You just have to figure out what's worth your fight. What lights you up? Who are you going to invest your love in? Once you figure that out, you can be truly free to be whoever you are and be the person you want to become in this life.

Birthdays

There is a moment during every delivery where time slows down and, for me, seems to stop. I have always found deliveries, cesarean sections, and surgeries to be my favorite part of my job. During those moments I can be more present and solely focused on one thing. If someone down the hallway needs me, I can't do it; I am delivering a baby. That being said, it's not like I turn off my brain, but in residency it seemed like those were the only times I was able to truly be present with the job I wanted to do for the rest of my life.

Every family has a story. Every person has his or her own challenges. I love being part of putting the puzzle together. Then, when the delivery day arrives, and the head emerges, either from a cesarean scar or vaginally from crowning, it's total wonder and joy that they get to have a new member of their family.

A few years ago, I had the privilege of taking care of a patient whom I admired a great deal. She and her family had been through a third trimester loss, still birth, because of various complications. She had many other pregnancy struggles as well. Sadly, some of these things are random and unpreventable and you can't do anything to see into the future and fix them.

She decided that instead of wallowing in sadness, she

was going to channel her son's energy into helping others. She became a bereavement doula to help parents who are struggling with current losses, but also to be an understanding ear when they get pregnant again. I think most people who have lost a baby, newborn, or child of any age live in a sense of worry that what they have currently can easily be taken away.

She decided to get pregnant again, and when she did, I was on her management team. She had a high-risk pregnancy for various reasons and needed titration of insulin for diabetes. At the end of the pregnancy, her insulin requirements started dropping, and of course, this prompted anxiety for her and the people who were caring for her as this seemed like the same story. In these cases, it could mean the placenta isn't working as efficiently as it needs to nourish the baby. At one point, she ceased needing insulin despite having significant needs immediately before.

The patient came in for monitoring at the office frequently. She had growth ultrasounds and biophysical profiles to make sure the baby was doing well. As one of the physicians who knew her and her story, I had a more heightened sense of awareness of what was going on in her pregnancy. My partner at the time would give me updates when I didn't see her, and we would talk through his thoughts. He knew I was the backup plan for delivery. After going through a trauma like she did, we wanted to make sure she was comfortable with everyone taking care of her and that we were all on the same page.

When her main doctor was gone or unavailable, we had this unspoken understanding that I would be there if she needed something. Of course, when he was out of town, I got a call from his nurse. She apologized as I wasn't on call, and the on-call doctor told her to monitor symptoms. She explained that the patient stopped needing insulin, she was contracting, uncomfortable, and pre-term at this time. I told her to go into the hospital, as I knew this would be an eerily similar story for her and likely cause a lot of anxiety.

I met her in triage so I could assess the data for myself. Physicians should never make decisions on emotion, even though it is hard to separate those feelings at times. While I was there, I realized she needed to be delivered. We went ahead with the cesarean section. We brought her into the operating room. In the operating room there is always a team present. The anesthesiologist and a CRNA are always up by the patient's head. There is a nurse for the patient and one for the baby. We have a surgical technician to help with the tools, suture, retract, create better visualization, and at times comic relief. In cases where we want to make sure the baby has more resources, we often will have the Neonatal Nurse Practitioner there as well.

I was standing outside the operating room scrubbing my hands for surgery and watching through the window to see how prep was going when time stopped. Nothing else matters except the patient and the fetus. You get a sense of calm because you know you're doing the right thing. After thousands of deliveries, you realize you can handle almost anything, and if you haven't seen it before, you have enough experience to get yourself out of the situation. For that strength, I really thank the toughness and constant chaos of residency. I think I had the best program for a general OBGYN.

When the patient is prepped, the timers go off, and the drapes are in place, we always do a time-out. Time-outs were created in medicine to make sure we have the right patient and we are doing the correct procedure. Cesareans, of course, are a little different because the patient is awake and can interact, however, it isn't treated any differently.

I watched a reality TV show about Lenox Hill Hospital during the pandemic. During timeouts they go around the room and say what each person is thankful for. I thought this seemed like an amazing way to start the day and have since tried to incorporate this into my timeouts. As a young female physician, there used to be people who intimidated me, however, you get over that quickly, especially if you talk about what you're thankful for.

In the OR we then test the patient to make sure she isn't in any pain. They bring the partner into the room and he or she can sit by the patient's head during the procedure. Some partners watch, some cry, some laugh, others sit and stare at the mother-to-be and can't imagine looking over the drape.

On this day, for this birthday, when I was able to bring her daughter into the world and be the first person to touch her little fuzzy hair, it gave me such a sense of relief, joy, and hope. When you do a cesarean for fetal indications, there is always a moment where you worry if things are going to be fine. As soon as she emerged, she was feisty and cried. Here was a little girl who was perfect, new, and entering into life with a clean slate. Mostly, for my part, I was happy she was safe, and I got to be there for her delivery. I looked at her and realized how hard her parents had fought for her to be with us, and it all made sense.

When we rolled the patient into the recovery area, she told me she knew I would come for the delivery, which seemed perplexing because I didn't know I would come on my day off when I wasn't her main doctor.

'I knew you wouldn't let him or me down,' she said with a smirk.

'You're right. Nowhere else I would rather be.' And I meant that.

That's what partners are for. You take care of each other's patients as if they're you're own because they are. You hope other people feel the same way about your patients when the time comes. Years later, the patient told me that she spoke with a medium when she was pregnant. The medium had told her that her primary physician wouldn't be able to be there, but I would be. So, she had no doubt how things would unfold. I realized then that we should all have more faith in each other and that things have an unusual way of working out.

Epilogue

I had a really hard time understanding how we could evolve into a situation where human life was deemed worthless. As a physician, my principles have always been unwavering. We, as physicians, don't pick and choose who we treat. We don't decide whose life is worth saving.

Watching a pandemic turn into a political circus was catastrophic to us. The community at large depends on accurate data from those in power and the medical communities nationally. If people can't trust that information, they will believe whatever fits the narrative they want to believe. Physicians understand that we can't provide medicine under the guidance of wishful thinking.

The great mask debate propelled us further into the black hole of misinformation. It also, extracted some of our humanity. When you look at a person, what do you see? I'm not talking during the pandemic; I am talking in the before times. During the beautiful pre-2020 era where you could walk around with your hair in a pony tail and nothing on your face, I usually notice someone's eyes and smile. Studies show smiling actually helps reduce stress for you and those in your proximity. Smiling helps you to form attachments with other people. Someone's ability to communicate with their face is critical to self-expression.

Now we are thrown into a polarized political upheaval

dealing with a pandemic, and we are unable to relate fully to others in our true humanity. With mask wearing however, you have the group that believe one set of scientific data and the group that follow something else. Those who wear masks become angry and frustrated with those that don't. Then there are people who opt do no research for themselves and are just angry that their lives are disrupted.

Recently, I went into the hospital for a delivery. My patient had been tested for COVID-19 on admission to the hospital, was negative. When I saw my patient, it was the first time, in her entire pregnancy, that I saw her face. In that moment, it dawned on me, that she had never seen mine. When we made jokes about pregnancy during prenatal appointments, she had never seen my smile. She probably even had a hard time making out the structure of my eyes behind the shield and the mask with the fluorescent light reflecting off the plastic. Despite the extra layers of the pandemic, she and I were able to bond, and find commonality in the chaos. The masks we wore, our outer layers, didn't mean anything about the people we are.

I also realized that race and gender, like masks, are the outer layer that often exists as an unnecessary barrier. These things shouldn't matter to how we are truly seen in the world. However, in this divisive climate, I think the focus is more on what we can see for ourselves, and not what we might hear third hand.

The most transformative moment of my life came in a meeting during which I was stripped of any humanity, dignity, integrity, and it was because I was a woman, and I had no power. My voice didn't matter. My contributions were mute. It was the external construct that allowed me to be debased in front of everyone. I was not allowed to have the same rights or treatment as others because of who I am.

When I started writing this book, I dedicated it, in part, to Ruth Bader Ginsberg. Now it is being dedicated to her in memoriam. She was an amazing advocate for women. We forget how little power we had before she took up the fight. When I am cast aside because of my gender, I remember the place in which she started. I live in amazement of the things she achieved. Sometimes, we need these transformative moments in our life, to teach us that we need to be our own heroes. That we need to fight for the things that are right in the world. That all men and women, regardless of sexuality or race, should be considered equal under the law. A democracy, is only just, when we treat everyone with equality, dignity, and respect.

'Speak your mind even if your voice shakes.' RBG

When I was writing, my daughter asked what I was working on. I told her I was writing a book. She smiled and asked, 'Does it have a happy ending?'

Well, that's the thing about the book of our life; we have the power to decide if it is going to have a happy ending or not. Each chapter might not end well, but the sum-total of who we are and what we can do as individuals can be inspiring, fierce, and happy. The beautiful thing is our stories aren't over, if we continue to write them.

When things are dark in our lives, we have choices. We can either quit, run away, die, or we can fight for what's important to us. There are many times I wanted to give up. There are days when I couldn't find the path forward, felt stuck and betrayed. I chose to fight. I have chosen to love people despite all the evidence that it could be challenging.

Write your own story! Love with your whole heart! Don't give up on yourself!